Puzzles for Medical Students:
Paediatrics

For Michael, my husband...

Puzzles for Medical Students: Paediatrics

Ranjita Howard MBChB BSc (Hons)
Managing Director, Medicas
www.medicas.org.uk

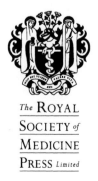

The ROYAL
SOCIETY of
MEDICINE
PRESS Limited

© 2008 Royal Society of Medicine Press Ltd

Published by the Royal Society of Medicine Press Ltd
1 Wimpole Street, London W1G 0AE, UK
Tel: +44 (0)20 7290 2921
Fax: +44 (0)20 7290 2929
Email: publishing@rsm.ac.uk
Website: www.rsmpress.co.uk

British Library Cataloguing in Publication Data
A catalogue record for this book is available from the British Library

ISBN 978-1-85315-791-2

Distribution in Europe and Rest of World:
Marston Book Services Ltd
PO Box 269
Abingdon
Oxon OX14 4YN, UK
Tel: +44 (0)1235 465500
Fax: +44 (0)1235 465555
Email: direct.order@marston.co.uk

Distribution in the USA and Canada:
Royal Society of Medicine Press Ltd
c/o BookMasters Inc
30 Amberwood Parkway
Ashland, OH 44805, USA
Tel: +1 800 247 6553/+1 800 266 5564
Fax: +1 419 281 6883
Email: orders@bookmasters.com

Distribution in Australia and New Zealand:
Elsevier Australia
30-52 Smidmore Street
Marrickville NSW 2204, Australia
Tel: +61 2 9517 8999
Fax: +61 2 9517 2249
Email: service@elsevier.com.au

Typeset by Phoenix Photosetting, Chatham, Kent
Printed in Europe by the Alden Group, Oxford

Contents

Foreword

There are many textbooks of medicine on today's market for medical students. However, *Puzzles for Medical Students* is something different – very different. Unlike bland medical textbooks offering learning by rote, Ranjita's book challenges the medical student to learn key medical facts through the novel approach of solving puzzles. The application of puzzle solving to medical education is new, which is surprising, as the benefits of word searching in education have been known for some time.

This book does not pretend to be a substitute medical textbook: this would be unrealistic. However, what this book does well is to supplement the classical didactic approach often witnessed at medical school.

Ultimately, it will provide the necessary variety for medical students to obviate fatigue, which is a common feature of those at a medical undergraduate level. Indeed, the purpose of the wordsearches is to provide a more fun and interactive way of remembering lists, whilst crosswords are aimed at testing specific knowledge in a relaxed, more familiar and exciting way. The answers are presented in tables to allow for conciseness and for ease of comparison. There are also helpful hints and tips throughout the book, highlighting areas of confusion alongside the clearly presented puzzles.

Enjoy your puzzle solving!

Andrew Catto BSc PhD MBChB FRCP
Consultant Physician, Airedale NHS Trust

Preface

The idea for writing this kind of book came to me during my final year at medical school. It was clear that other than through the use of textbooks and conventional lecturing methods, there was little variety in the way one learned and revised such a broad and vast a subject as medicine. The reason why I chose word puzzles was twofold. First of all, despite their worldwide popularity and obvious educational benefits, word puzzles have yet to be fully utilized as an educational tool, particularly as it applies to medical students. Second, given the obvious dryness of textbook learning, my intentions were to help liberalize the learning process through making it lighter, more fun and less fatiguing. Indeed, the use of puzzles can divert the attention of medical students away from the pressures of medical school in favour of a mental state that is more relaxed and therefore more productive cognitively.

To use the wordsearches, I would suggest you first write down a list of potential differential causes, and then search for them in the relevant grid. If you do not manage to remember all those required, then a scan over the grid may jog your memory. The use of crosswords, on the other hand, is self-explanatory, and they will go a long way towards testing you on key information that you should know as a potential doctor. However, do not feel too alarmed if you cannot get all the clues, as this book challenges one's knowledge of both common and less common diagnoses. What you will find is that the tables accompanying the answers are formatted and structured in a way that assists the long-term recall of even the most difficult of subjects.

There are a number ways that you can use this book. For example, when you are on your paediatric placement and you are faced with a case of a recurrent cough, you can subsequently turn to this section of the book to progressively challenge and clarify your understanding of differential diagnosis as it applies to this subject. Indeed, it is most effective to pull this book out from your bag immediately after seeing a clinical case and challenge yourself straight away. Secondly, you may choose to test yourself on specific topics that you are perhaps having difficulty with, and use the tables accompanying the answers to fill any knowledge gaps you may have. Alternatively, the book can simply be used to test yourself randomly on different subjects throughout your paediatric syllabus.

However, I feel this book is at its most useful when coming up to your examinations, because during those long hours of tedious revision, this book will provide a brief respite and light relief with its more informal delivery.

I hope you enjoy using this book and that it will go some way towards helping you pass your paediatric examinations, albeit with a lighter and more refreshing tone!

Ranjita Howard

PUZZLES

1. Nutrition

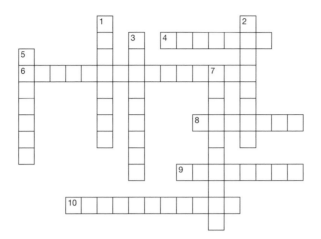

Across

4 Component of cow's milk present at much higher level than in human milk (7)

6 Immunity provided through breast milk (14,1)

8 Term for the baby eating solid food as opposed to only breast milk (7)

9 Congenital defect in babies that prevents them from being able to suckle (5,3)

10 Malnutrition disorder in which the child is fed on a diet high in starch but low in protein (11)

Down

1 Anti-infective enzyme in breast milk (8)

2 If deficient, can cause eye disease (7,1)

3 Yellow fluid secreted from the breast in the first days after delivery (9)

5 Vitamin D deficiency (7)

7 Component of breast milk that has antiviral properties (10)

2. Causes of Vomiting

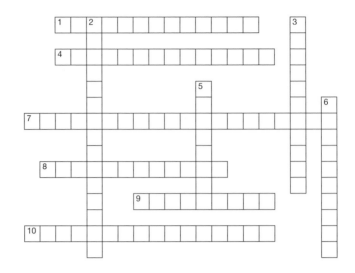

Across

1 Metabolic cause of vomiting (13)
4 Self-induced vomiting (7,7)
7 Obstruction of the large intestine in neonates (13,7)
8 Central abdominal pain associated with vomiting in children over 2 years of age (12)
9 Regurgitation of small amount of milk post-feeding (9)
10 Anatomical structure, if incompetent, results in gastro-oesophageal reflux (7,9)

Down

2 Projectile, non-bilious vomiting in babies 4–8 years old (7,8)
3 Must be considered in gastroenteritis (11)
5 Visual disturbances preceding chronic unilateral headaches and recurrent vomiting (8)
6 Disease of nervous system in which acute vomiting is a symptom (10)

3. Acute Abdominal Pain

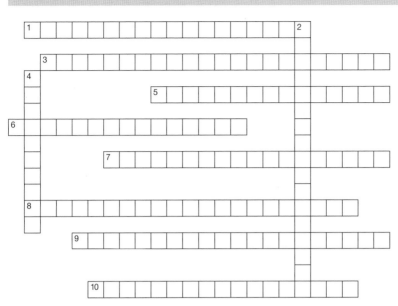

Across

1 Medical cause of referred abdominal pain associated with chest pain and purulent sputum (5,4,9)

3 Child with joint pain, purpuric rash and colicky abdominal pain (6-9,7)

5 Baby with episodic, colicky pain and 'redcurrant jelly' stools noticed on rectal examination (15)

6 Abdominal pain with diarrhoea and vomiting (15)

7 Right iliac fossa pain with recent history of upper respiratory tract infection (10,8)

8 Cause of acute, central abdominal pain with a history of excessive rectal bleeding, in children under 10 years old (7,14)

9 Acute abdominal pain with slow, deep breathing and distinctive odour on the breath (8,12)

10 Painful scrotal swelling with pain radiating upwards towards the abdomen (10,7)

Down

2 Child presenting with anorexia, low-grade fever and central, colicky pain which has migrated to the right iliac fossa (5,12)

4 Surgical intervention to diagnose acute cause of abdominal pain and peritonism (10)

4. Causes of Recurrent Abdominal Pain

Find 18 causes of recurrent abdominal pain in the grid. Words can go horizontally, vertically and diagonally in all eight directions.

C	M	A	L	R	O	T	A	T	I	O	N	T	P	X	R	Z	H	T	L	L	M	P	L	E
B	A	T	G	R	T	Q	T	Q	R	L	R	E	B	L	K	L	F	G	B	X	L	G	V	S
N	L	L	V	C	M	M	M	L	K	T	P	C	O	N	S	T	I	P	A	T	I	O	N	A
Y	O	D	C	N	V	Y	C	T	D	T	G	N	R	M	E	Y	T	F	W	G	Q	C	T	E
D	R	I	B	U	P	R	W	V	I	L	N	M	L	R	M	C	M	Q	R	I	Y	L	Q	S
M	W	R	T	F	L	R	X	C	L	R	J	H	B	B	O	C	R	D	U	A	G	N	X	I
Q	L	N	L	P	T	U	U	N	R	H	B	K	G	D	R	Y	F	S	O	R	G	O	Z	D
D	L	P	D	W	E	L	S	H	L	M	T	S	Q	C	D	E	T	I	M	D	L	N	Y	Y
S	J	C	Y	B	C	C	H	R	G	G	I	B	R	J	N	X	H	T	U	I	N	U	R	R
D	I	P	R	E	P	P	S	L	N	T	N	Q	Y	I	Y	M	X	I	T	A	R	L	T	O
Z	K	T	R	O	F	N	T	U	I	T	Q	P	A	M	S	L	G	T	N	S	L	C	P	T
L	G	L	I	H	H	Q	X	R	S	G	N	R	M	K	L	N	R	A	A	I	C	E	P	A
X	K	B	N	T	X	N	T	B	M	S	G	L	T	H	E	K	V	E	I	S	R	R	W	M
W	L	N	K	L	A	S	S	L	D	I	U	V	F	T	W	P	K	R	R	L	L	D	C	M
P	Q	L	N	Y	A	P	T	D	M	V	B	T	B	R	O	N	V	C	A	X	L	Y	N	A
P	N	P	K	G	L	K	E	L	I	T	D	J	N	R	B	L	T	N	V	Q	W	S	Z	L
D	L	M	P	M	T	B	A	H	Q	S	N	V	P	I	E	X	X	A	O	G	K	P	C	F
P	L	R	L	G	H	N	R	W	J	C	E	H	H	H	L	V	Q	P	T	V	G	E	Y	N
L	L	R	N	D	I	Y	V	R	K	M	Y	A	N	X	B	F	J	R	J	P	D	P	T	I
M	J	T	F	M	C	R	F	M	R	R	Z	V	S	M	A	P	J	X	K	L	W	S	X	C
Z	M	V	O	K	H	M	Q	Q	I	F	T	K	V	E	T	V	V	B	F	H	B	I	C	I
B	W	D	W	R	L	P	J	A	Q	T	R	L	B	X	I	K	H	Y	N	Y	P	A	T	V
N	B	T	N	O	I	T	C	E	F	N	I	T	C	A	R	T	Y	R	A	N	I	R	U	L
A	K	J	Y	C	N	R	D	H	L	D	N	Z	W	R	R	T	K	X	Z	Y	N	C	Y	E
V	S	I	T	I	T	S	Y	C	E	L	O	H	C	F	I	T	N	X	P	M	G	C	J	P

5. Causes of Constipation

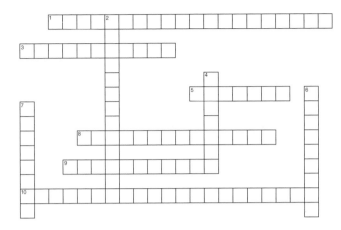

Across

1 History of delayed passage of meconium and distended abdomen that appears empty on examination (13,7)
3 Congenital absence of anal orifice (4,7)
5 Constipation with overflow (7)
8 Systemic cause of chronic constipation (14)
9 Hard, impacted stools may cause this (4,7)
10 Chronic obstruction of the bowel may predispose to this by mere proximity (7,5,9)

Down

2 Neurological disorder with features of constipation (8,5)
4 Medication with an adverse effect of constipation (7)
6 Acute constipation post-surgery (9)
7 Twisting of the bowel resulting in intestinal obstruction (8)

6. Causes of Chronic Diarrhoea

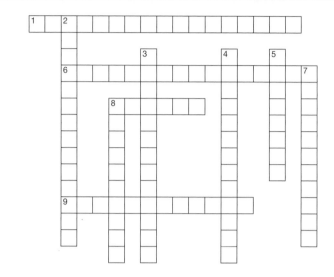

Across

1 Chronic disorder with the presentation of diarrhoea with blood and mucus (10,7)

6 Frequent episodes of passing undigested food in preschoolers (7,9)

8 Substance that patients with coeliac disease are sensitive to (6)

9 Type of stools seen in coeliac disease (12)

Down

2 Chronic diarrhoea along with recurrent lung infections (6,7)

3 Diagnosis to confirm coeliac disease (7,6)

4 Episodes of abdominal pain, diarrhoea, delayed puberty along with perianal ulcers; starts in adolescence (6,7)

5 Allergy to a particular food which results in vomiting and diarrhoea (4,4)

7 Type of antibody to screen for coeliac disease (11)

8 Persistent passage of fatty pale stools after returning from abroad (10)

7. Gastroenteritis

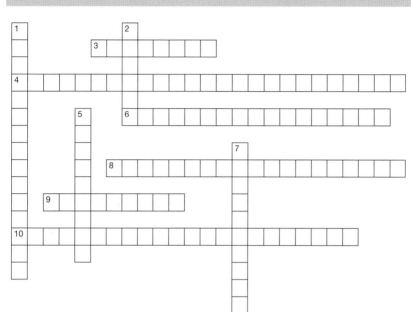

Across

3 Pathogen causing symptoms of bloody stools with pus, fever and, in some cases, febrile convulsions (8)

4 Microangiopathic haemolyitc anaemia, thrombocytopenia and acute renal failure following gastrointestinal infection (10,7,8)

6 Sign of moderate to severe dehydration (7,4,6)

8 Severe abdominal pain and bloody diarrhoea when ingesting this bacterium in contaminated chicken or milk (13,6)

9 Most common cause of gastroenteritis in the developed world (9)

10 Main form of management for mild dehydration (4,11,7)

Down

1 Causes watery diarrhoea with vomiting after consuming undercooked meat (11,4)

2 Most common time of year that 9 *Across* is spread (6)

5 Term for severe diarrhoea with blood and mucus (9)

7 Bacteria ingested through undercooked eggs (10)

8. Causes of Rectal Bleeding

Find 17 causes of rectal bleeding in the grid. Words can go horizontally, vertically and diagonally in all eight directions.

N	H	W	Y	L	T	H	N	V	J	M	Q	T	H	J	V	N	R	Y	T	T	N	K	T	V
E	E	X	M	V	N	A	K	T	P	Q	M	P	K	C	K	M	R	N	T	R	Z	J	C	K
N	N	K	G	T	N	E	V	N	D	P	C	L	T	T	L	B	L	Q	F	K	B	D	T	T
T	O	Q	W	T	Z	M	U	L	U	C	I	T	R	E	V	I	D	S	L	E	K	C	E	M
A	C	R	X	M	M	O	Z	E	G	C	F	Z	W	Q	T	W	M	B	J	F	R	Y	V	H
M	H	I	Z	N	K	L	F	Q	R	G	D	P	S	E	X	U	A	L	A	B	U	S	E	A
E	S	N	V	L	P	Y	Q	R	B	U	Z	Y	G	X	P	B	W	T	A	R	X	G	M	E
O	C	U	Y	L	Y	T	P	N	A	N	S	Y	K	Y	M	L	N	L	E	T	V	J	H	M
B	H	J	B	N	N	I	W	L	L	M	L	S	Z	G	K	K	L	C	R	X	M	C	S	O
A	O	E	L	O	R	C	X	L	L	W	M	B	I	N	Z	E	T	X	H	Q	T	I	W	R
H	N	J	Y	I	Q	U	R	Q	E	K	J	T	D	F	N	A	R	W	H	D	T	H	M	R
I	L	R	C	T	Z	R	W	D	G	M	K	K	M	O	L	P	Z	K	F	I	V	V	Y	H
S	E	E	T	P	V	A	N	T	I	Q	M	Q	M	P	Z	A	R	M	L	Z	L	N	J	O
T	I	T	J	E	Y	E	T	B	H	T	Z	L	O	L	R	G	N	O	P	M	W	X	K	I
O	N	C	R	C	G	M	T	X	S	R	A	L	M	G	N	X	C	A	L	N	F	F	T	D
L	P	A	Z	S	R	I	Z	R	P	S	Y	M	T	R	C	E	R	G	W	A	G	T	G	S
Y	U	B	M	U	E	C	Q	R	T	P	Z	G	R	F	V	T	N	P	L	Y	P	M	N	D
T	R	O	M	S	L	S	C	R	O	H	N	S	D	I	S	E	A	S	E	K	M	S	R	L
I	P	L	T	S	L	Y	M	K	X	H	Q	R	T	J	L	F	M	Y	Y	X	N	P	E	R
C	U	Y	X	U	A	N	L	N	W	G	B	A	F	B	D	C	T	W	J	L	H	D	H	W
A	R	P	Q	T	K	D	C	N	R	L	R	W	D	P	Y	M	V	R	K	V	Y	C	Q	L
J	A	M	N	N	L	R	N	D	T	E	Y	P	K	F	G	F	B	M	A	M	Z	F	V	P
G	R	A	Q	I	I	O	W	X	C	C	N	D	R	X	K	Y	K	T	M	U	R	Q	Q	M
F	T	C	C	Y	M	M	Z	L	K	H	R	T	L	N	V	P	D	X	T	W	M	Z	K	Z
H	K	J	T	R	K	E	U	R	V	Q	L	K	M	W	T	W	T	T	N	M	Y	A	B	C

9. Genital Disorders

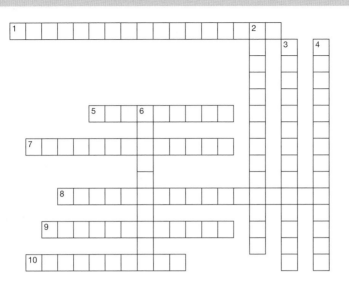

Across

1 Cause of no testis being present in the scrotum (11,6)
5 Painless scrotal swelling that transilluminates in the darkness (9)
7 Testis cannot be manipulated into scrotum (7,6)
8 Acute pain in the scrotum, groin and lower abdomen (10,7)
9 Inability to retract prepuce over the glans penis (12)
10 Enlarged veins in scrotum (10)

Down

2 Scrotal swelling increases in size on coughing (8,6)
3 Term encapsulating *1 Across* and *7 Across* (14)
4 Pain in the vulva associated with vaginal discharge (14)
6 Impalpable testis in scrotum can be massaged into scrotum when child is in squatting position, but returns to original position (10)

10. Renal Disease

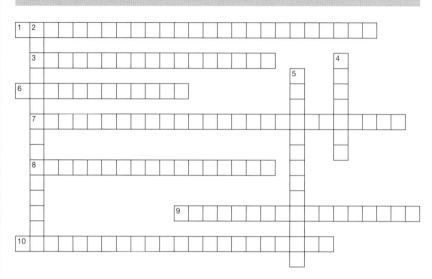

Across

1 Renal failure following a gastrointestinal infection (10,7,8)
3 Facial swelling in *9 Across* and *8 Across* (11,6)
6 Treatment for *8 Across* (12)
7 Rare vasculitic cause of *9 Across* (8,5,13)
8 Hypoalbuminaemia, proteinuria and generalised oedema (9,8)
9 Glomerulonephritis with characteristic oedema, hypertension and haematuria (9,8)
10 Glomerulonephritis with symmetrical rash and joint pain (6-9,7)

Down

2 Familial disorder which can lead to chronic renal failure and deafness (7,8)
4 Significant swelling in *8 Across* (7)
5 Infective organism that often causes nephritic syndrome (13)

11. Urinary Tract Infections

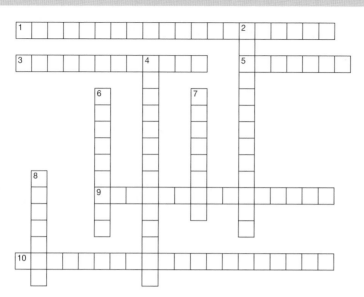

Across

1 Predisposing congenital abnormality in which urine returns from the bladder to the ureter (14,6)

3 First line of treatment (12)

5 Dipsticks test for this to check for bacteria in the urine (7)

9 Most likely bacterial cause (11,4)

10 Procedure to obtain urine sample in a baby (10,10)

Down

2 Possible sequelae of UTIs (5,8)

4 Symptoms of UTIs combined with loin pain (14)

6 Collecting an uncontaminated urine sample in older children (9)

7 Lower UTI symptoms without systemic features (8)

8 Pathogen affecting boys more than girls (7)

12. Causes of Haematuria

Find 18 causes of haematuria in the grid. Words can go horizontally, vertically and diagonally in all eight directions.

H	H	N	N	S	H	D	B	R	A	L	P	O	R	T	S	S	Y	N	D	R	O	M	E	Q	P
A	M	J	W	Y	W	F	P	X	T	M	L	L	L	X	Q	B	H	K	V	W	W	R	Y	M	K
E	K	W	Q	S	N	N	J	G	R	Z	D	K	N	K	B	X	G	N	J	P	H	K	G	E	W
M	P	A	T	T	S	T	T	M	T	T	K	C	Y	R	D	K	N	F	M	T	X	M	D	T	J
O	O	R	T	E	I	N	R	G	L	O	M	E	R	U	L	O	N	E	P	H	R	I	T	I	S
L	L	U	G	M	S	O	L	Y	R	T	W	R	T	H	H	R	Z	F	Z	R	M	K	M	T	D
Y	Y	P	C	I	O	I	P	D	K	W	N	M	N	J	W	B	C	F	L	A	V	M	G	K	Z
T	C	R	D	C	B	T	L	E	Q	T	M	Z	B	P	P	J	H	H	H	B	K	H	N	T	K
I	Y	U	K	L	M	C	R	X	M	N	M	N	K	Z	R	F	N	P	P	A	K	Q	T	A	K
C	S	P	L	U	O	E	H	E	R	W	C	Y	X	N	L	M	S	Z	N	H	R	T	I	J	Z
U	T	N	C	P	R	F	Z	R	W	J	H	B	H	A	V	O	R	T	X	T	T	N	M	P	K
R	I	I	K	U	H	N	K	C	T	T	G	Y	M	T	H	B	I	K	N	D	E	W	Q	H	T
A	C	E	J	S	T	I	Z	I	B	F	R	U	P	P	A	C	N	L	R	P	G	L	Y	W	B
E	K	L	K	E	R	T	T	S	T	D	A	C	O	E	O	P	C	X	O	M	K	W	W	W	P
M	I	N	L	R	A	C	X	E	X	R	J	L	S	A	R	M	O	T	M	V	B	V	L	Z	N
I	D	O	G	Y	L	A	L	M	T	N	C	F	G	T	W	C	Y	R	T	L	D	B	V	Y	J
C	N	H	R	T	U	R	M	D	M	Y	K	U	N	I	O	C	A	X	H	F	L	J	T	D	R
S	E	C	N	H	C	T	T	L	C	J	L	K	L	M	O	N	M	L	N	P	L	N	J	Z	Q
Y	Y	S	B	E	S	Y	C	Y	R	A	D	M	P	B	Y	J	E	Q	C	H	E	H	P	T	R
N	D	H	F	M	A	R	J	R	N	Q	S	N	M	Q	N	R	R	S	T	I	W	N	Q	P	T
D	I	C	F	A	V	A	X	T	G	T	T	O	M	L	L	C	K	K	Z	Q	U	M	A	M	R
R	S	O	T	T	L	N	S	K	U	F	R	C	B	W	M	W	M	L	N	N	M	R	T	G	M
O	E	N	T	O	A	I	Y	M	N	H	G	F	K	T	C	L	G	M	K	G	C	K	I	J	I
M	A	E	C	S	N	R	O	W	T	D	J	Q	L	R	G	W	K	T	M	N	C	B	L	A	Q
E	S	H	G	U	E	U	A	I	M	E	A	N	A	L	L	E	C	E	L	K	C	I	S	Z	T
W	E	T	L	S	R	M	L	R	R	Y	W	V	F	L	F	Q	Z	M	K	V	G	M	M	D	D

13. Causes of Acute Renal Failure

Find 16 causes of acute renal failure in the grid. Words can go horizontally, vertically and diagonally in all eight directions.

E	M	O	R	D	N	Y	S	S	S	E	R	T	S	I	D	Y	R	O	T	A	R	I	P	S	E	R
M	D	Q	R	D	R	Y	T	X	X	F	F	N	V	G	L	Z	T	B	G	D	T	X	F	Z	N	Q
Q	E	M	O	R	D	N	Y	S	C	I	M	E	A	R	U	C	I	T	Y	L	O	M	E	A	H	R
V	N	S	K	N	F	V	K	Y	D	C	Y	W	W	F	T	K	Q	Y	W	M	Z	D	H	M	L	V
X	K	L	I	K	P	D	K	L	R	J	F	C	N	F	D	H	X	M	H	X	V	H	F	M	P	Z
P	L	K	Z	S	P	V	L	K	N	L	M	K	R	C	K	N	W	M	B	C	L	Q	N	P	K	G
V	N	F	T	Q	O	T	W	K	N	Q	D	E	H	Y	D	R	A	T	I	O	N	S	P	V	Z	L
M	J	N	M	D	C	R	K	Q	Z	M	F	P	N	K	V	K	N	W	H	R	I	T	T	F	R	O
Y	D	Y	M	F	S	H	C	R	N	T	G	F	Q	M	L	C	H	T	C	T	K	P	K	E	Q	M
R	X	R	F	E	W	E	M	E	L	K	W	A	J	Z	M	X	X	B	I	Z	A	P	N	F	W	E
T	E	E	F	C	R	R	P	P	N	M	W	Z	S	Q	M	R	Q	R	F	P	V	A	P	N	W	R
T	M	N	G	X	G	U	V	S	V	R	D	G	W	T	W	F	H	C	I	N	L	G	E	D	D	U
M	O	A	H	L	T	L	L	K	I	K	A	G	H	K	R	P	Z	L	T	V	V	G	X	T	M	L
L	R	L	M	K	M	K	G	I	T	S	L	L	K	D	E	O	L	V	E	N	A	J	Y	Y	R	O
Y	D	C	Z	X	M	J	M	X	A	T	P	G	U	N	L	A	E	I	Z	H	Z	V	C	F	N	N
L	N	A	J	B	Y	W	V	B	R	F	V	N	O	B	R	W	N	N	R	M	R	L	N	K	S	E
F	Y	L	C	N	W	T	T	N	C	C	T	L	B	Y	U	T	Y	R	T	T	L	M	J	M	N	P
Y	S	C	G	M	K	C	P	H	L	Z	E	R	N	K	H	T	O	Z	V	E	Z	Z	C	R	R	H
N	C	U	Y	Q	B	L	T	R	T	Y	Q	E	A	R	M	M	E	M	X	N	R	F	R	K	U	R
Z	I	L	K	Y	T	N	Z	V	P	V	C	P	O	E	E	T	Z	T	T	T	B	I	Z	P	B	I
Q	T	I	L	H	D	N	K	Y	G	R	N	M	R	A	H	B	T	M	U	T	Y	F	T	R	F	T
M	O	M	V	H	V	K	K	N	O	G	B	D	H	Z	K	T	L	W	R	C	Y	D	H	I	R	I
W	R	G	G	L	M	T	N	S	T	O	X	H	K	W	V	R	W	Q	B	L	A	F	V	K	S	S
Y	H	R	X	F	L	W	I	K	S	X	Y	Y	T	K	Z	H	V	D	Y	G	T	Q	F	N	Q	N
G	P	P	T	K	X	S	R	I	L	J	R	W	M	Q	R	R	L	L	F	C	D	L	T	W	C	G
B	E	H	Z	N	L	L	S	R	W	M	L	L	R	L	Z	M	H	T	B	N	J	R	L	M	K	M
R	N	H	I	N	T	E	R	S	T	I	T	I	A	L	N	E	P	H	R	I	T	I	S	N	R	F

14. Headaches

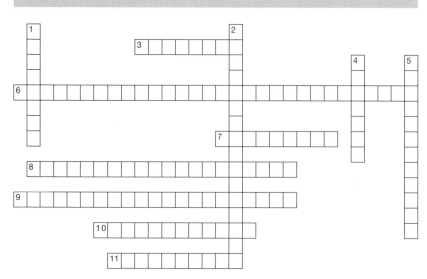

Across

3 Unilateral headache with preceding visual aura and nausea (8)

6 Throbbing headache with papilloedema in overweight female adolescents (6,12,12)

7 Headache combined with facial pain and rhinorrhoea (9)

8 Visual hallucination experienced in migraine (13,7)

9 Headache precipitated by mastication (17,4)

10 Rare cause but must be checked for (12)

11 Serious cause of headache and photophobia (10)

Down

1 Recreational drugs taken mainly by teenage boys in which headaches are a side effect (8)

2 They cause headache accompanied by blurry vision which can be rectified by prescriptive glasses (10,6)

4 Band-like headache associated with fatigue (7)

5 Headache along with tooth sensitivity when consuming hot or cold food (6,6)

15. Causes of Funny Turns

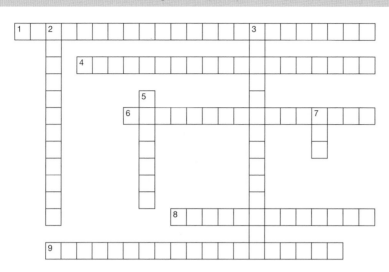

Across

1 Episodes of imbalance, nausea and nystagmus whilst remaining alert (6,10,7)

4 Crying toddler becomes silent and apnoeic with skin turning blue (6-7,6)

6 Deep breathing resulting in light-headedness along with tingling in hands, feet and lips (16)

8 Episodes of twitching with unconsciousness similar to that in epilepsy (13)

9 Preschooler becomes pale and loses consciousness, which may lead to tonic–clonic seizure (6,6,7)

Down

2 Whilst sleeping, toddler sits up with dilated pupils looking frightened (5,7)

3 A rare cardiac cause of fainting after exercise in adolescents (4,2,8)

5 Fainting in older children when standing for long periods (7)

7 Sudden involuntary movement (3)

16. Causes of Hearing Impairment

Find 16 causes of hearing impairment in the grid. Words can go horizontally, vertically and diagonally in all eight directions.

R	N	H	T	Z	H	Y	N	M	T	Y	M	R	L	R	G	P	K	X	T	X	F	E
Z	J	F	S	U	R	I	V	O	L	A	G	E	M	O	T	Y	C	R	P	D	Q	M
Q	P	O	F	G	M	A	Z	L	F	K	N	R	C	N	P	L	L	F	K	C	L	O
Q	V	R	Y	M	D	I	R	Y	W	R	K	K	R	H	F	N	X	B	Q	N	D	R
P	B	E	T	Z	H	D	G	J	T	F	N	Q	Q	M	R	F	X	Y	D	N	E	D
R	D	I	I	M	S	E	D	I	S	O	C	Y	L	G	O	N	I	M	A	N	M	N
L	B	G	R	T	M	M	F	D	F	D	K	T	Y	M	R	Q	H	G	C	Z	T	Y
V	W	N	U	N	M	S	W	C	O	L	Z	L	R	U	A	T	J	E	D	W	P	S
R	V	B	T	L	B	I	G	Q	L	W	L	W	B	Y	Z	L	P	D	A	F	L	S
Z	C	O	A	Q	V	T	L	R	M	T	N	E	H	Y	F	H	L	I	M	S	X	N
T	H	D	M	X	L	I	L	L	Y	B	L	S	T	R	A	K	X	E	U	T	Y	I
C	H	Y	E	F	K	T	J	R	H	L	D	G	S	L	W	Y	D	R	B	L	F	L
P	C	T	R	C	Z	O	R	D	A	L	C	N	I	Y	H	Q	E	Z	L	U	X	L
H	W	N	P	L	X	Y	R	V	T	P	D	T	F	P	N	T	D	C	H	F	R	O
C	M	W	J	E	G	R	V	L	N	W	I	T	S	R	C	D	L	T	N	T	M	C
T	Z	M	L	F	Z	O	Y	Q	N	S	A	A	N	I	X	X	R	W	R	Y	W	R
N	B	W	M	T	N	T	J	D	P	B	H	X	N	J	T	J	M	O	X	W	T	E
K	V	D	T	P	C	E	D	N	Y	T	T	R	X	W	V	D	P	K	M	T	K	H
C	N	M	K	A	T	R	H	K	R	R	E	P	H	T	L	H	D	W	C	E	J	C
K	X	K	N	L	T	C	M	I	N	K	D	Q	J	L	T	W	T	B	J	C	P	A
W	N	L	R	A	N	E	B	N	N	K	D	Q	T	T	Q	N	T	K	T	R	B	E
K	Z	K	Q	T	L	S	M	E	N	I	N	G	I	T	I	S	V	J	F	G	T	R
R	X	V	N	E	V	D	O	T	O	S	C	L	E	R	O	S	I	S	T	P	T	T

17. Bacterial Meningitis

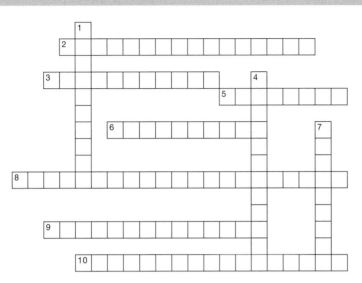

Across

2 Main antibiotic if *Neisseria meningitidis* is isolated (16)

3 Sign described by older children (11)

5 Serious complication if not appropriately treated (8)

6 Sign suggestive of neck stiffness (10)

8 Infective agent in neonates (8,13)

9 Investigation to identify aetiology (6,8)

10 Late sign in babies (7,10)

Down

1 Antibiotic treating a range of bacteria (10)

4 If sign present, investigation (lumbar) should not be performed (12)

7 Type of meningococcal rash (9)

18. Causes of Learning Disabilities

Find 16 causes of learning disabilities in the grid. Words can go horizontally, vertically and diagonally in all eight directions.

T	T	J	K	M	T	L	B	V	M	R	D	J	W	N	T	G	B	P	K	R	Z	R	L	M	C	K	D	K	L
R	T	Y	Y	G	W	T	R	G	M	Z	K	Y	K	N	R	L	A	N	N	H	T	H	V	T	M	R	J	J	V
Y	J	G	K	D	E	B	G	L	T	R	B	R	F	K	Y	B	J	L	M	G	P	R	F	N	T	X	N	H	B
N	P	R	G	D	M	M	L	T	G	N	B	T	K	W	W	L	Y	J	A	T	J	M	L	K	N	X	N	V	M
D	T	H	P	W	O	B	O	R	L	H	Q	M	L	D	G	T	J	R	Z	C	N	Y	A	R	G	T	Y	R	N
D	N	N	K	M	R	P	J	R	C	H	E	A	D	I	N	J	U	R	Y	W	T	L	D	T	P	K	L	N	L
T	M	P	G	S	D	Z	R	N	D	R	N	V	Z	L	J	T	R	L	Y	K	L	O	K	N	W	N	N	R	B
T	Q	F	H	U	N	Y	Q	P	Z	N	M	T	F	W	Q	X	K	Z	R	E	W	T	S	P	G	G	T	J	R
E	L	L	N	R	Y	Y	C	C	M	T	Y	V	P	K	X	K	F	H	B	F	D	N	R	A	T	R	M	N	M
M	K	W	E	I	S	N	Y	W	K	Q	Y	S	L	E	K	N	Q	U	T	W	G	T	K	L	E	C	C	P	R
O	C	R	U	V	S	T	N	C	G	R	M	M	L	K	Q	C	R	R	C	B	M	N	Y	N	C	M	M	J	J
R	K	Y	R	O	R	V	R	B	E	M	M	I	L	O	D	M	X	P	M	L	N	X	K	W	V	Q	I	L	R
D	L	T	O	L	E	R	T	T	M	C	G	M	L	Q	H	Q	F	E	L	M	T	D	L	R	B	L	R	A	B
N	P	Y	F	A	T	B	R	M	O	A	N	L	M	N	Q	O	N	K	H	Y	X	R	P	H	P	H	K	M	T
Y	T	T	I	G	L	J	Y	D	R	R	R	Q	E	T	J	I	C	P	P	C	J	N	J	V	T	Y	H	J	N
S	Z	T	B	E	E	Z	M	F	D	T	Q	N	Q	A	N	W	X	L	M	T	L	T	B	L	J	P	F	M	R
I	Z	J	R	M	F	D	Y	X	N	G	H	Q	T	G	D	W	Q	T	A	W	N	Q	B	R	R	O	W	P	W
L	K	Q	O	O	E	L	D	Y	Y	N	Q	K	I	V	W	P	K	Z	Q	L	L	T	Y	P	H	G	V	L	R
L	N	N	M	T	N	M	M	M	S	P	Z	T	T	W	V	K	O	N	V	P	A	B	G	L	W	L	M	T	K
I	T	T	A	Y	I	G	H	L	S	N	I	H	T	K	D	R	L	I	D	T	J	T	K	K	T	Y	D	Z	M
W	D	V	T	C	L	F	K	L	N	S	N	Q	M	P	W	H	X	N	S	J	K	Z	E	D	T	C	T	N	M
R	C	J	O	X	K	W	L	P	W	Y	C	L	V	B	H	V	R	D	R	O	R	R	Y	F	T	A	R	L	J
E	T	F	S	P	T	T	P	C	O	H	Z	P	R	K	J	Q	K	G	T	P	N	X	G	R	O	E	T	V	C
D	V	Q	I	N	K	X	K	C	D	Z	V	H	K	F	X	Q	M	V	F	Y	H	I	R	R	Q	M	N	V	C
A	L	M	S	B	L	E	M	O	R	D	N	Y	S	S	T	T	E	R	T	L	N	C	N	W	H	I	V	W	K
R	L	W	T	H	N	N	L	M	Q	M	Y	X	T	L	H	L	W	H	R	Z	B	N	D	G	K	A	W	J	B
P	T	C	L	P	J	P	H	E	N	Y	L	K	E	T	O	N	U	R	I	A	R	N	H	C	Y	B	N	R	Y
H	Y	P	O	X	I	C	I	S	C	H	A	E	M	I	C	E	N	C	E	P	H	A	L	O	P	A	T	H	Y
T	C	V	D	T	J	V	K	N	H	G	H	W	F	H	X	L	L	Q	K	C	M	Q	F	T	W	V	T	Z	D
V	W	T	K	M	K	G	M	B	L	T	M	L	L	P	N	K	Y	R	C	V	N	L	Y	W	Q	T	Q	M	V

19. Causes of Cerebral Palsy

Find 15 causes of cerebral palsy in the grid. Words can go horizontally, vertically and diagonally in all eight directions.

N	J	X	F	P	D	Q	K	Q	M	N	Y	F	D	H	Y	D	R	O	C	E	P	H	A	L	U	S	X	Y	B
H	R	H	L	L	G	B	Y	N	M	X	B	J	Q	T	W	R	B	N	Q	L	B	R	P	D	E	K	X	H	F
N	Y	L	Y	H	C	N	L	Q	C	T	Y	F	J	T	C	L	T	S	V	B	B	X	G	Z	G	H	W	T	D
M	C	P	N	R	N	C	W	F	H	M	K	G	N	K	R	T	U	Q	R	L	N	R	V	N	A	N	W	A	M
C	B	L	E	J	K	L	M	K	N	M	W	Z	T	Q	Y	R	G	K	T	Y	J	N	G	W	H	F	J	P	B
B	C	H	Y	R	R	R	L	W	M	Z	H	R	P	B	I	K	A	L	M	F	X	N	C	F	R	L	N	O	T
Q	C	N	Q	L	B	R	L	L	H	J	R	C	T	V	R	I	Q	K	N	Y	K	T	N	B	R	N	M	L	T
D	G	E	K	P	W	I	L	R	J	L	T	J	O	N	M	W	X	M	K	V	G	R	R	T	O	J	R	A	R
K	C	T	R	F	M	N	L	K	B	G	R	L	Q	E	V	P	C	H	V	L	Y	K	L	C	M	L	T	H	L
V	N	Y	C	E	D	L	K	I	P	M	A	H	A	P	H	N	Z	P	Z	C	G	D	R	M	E	T	N	P	R
N	O	R	M	W	B	X	B	K	R	G	Q	C	F	W	Z	N	G	W	N	Z	X	L	H	D	A	R	M	E	W
T	N	K	Z	M	L	R	T	M	E	U	Y	L	S	I	T	I	L	A	H	P	E	C	N	E	H	T	D	C	J
L	A	C	V	X	M	F	A	M	Z	L	B	N	J	T	B	R	B	M	Q	M	V	V	V	T	R	T	C	N	C
H	C	F	B	K	K	W	O	L	G	L	N	I	Q	F	Y	R	L	T	T	J	T	P	M	J	A	F	J	E	B
T	C	W	I	L	B	T	X	O	D	V	V	T	N	H	D	J	R	N	N	V	K	T	J	L	L	T	W	C	B
B	I	J	R	W	Y	T	P	P	Z	Y	K	Q	Y	A	Q	R	Z	X	X	T	W	C	H	K	U	H	G	I	I
K	D	F	T	C	T	Y	M	H	H	R	S	Z	T	M	E	T	B	L	H	M	N	T	F	N	C	D	T	M	R
P	E	V	H	H	H	L	X	H	N	X	B	G	R	B	T	M	R	B	K	Z	K	L	N	Z	I	V	K	E	T
X	N	D	I	F	Q	G	C	L	P	D	Y	W	E	K	Z	L	I	L	T	H	K	L	T	T	R	Y	D	A	H
R	T	T	N	N	V	T	H	D	X	J	Y	M	C	N	F	T	G	A	K	N	B	W	A	T	T	M	T	H	A
T	A	D	J	L	M	V	T	G	B	P	E	R	N	Q	E	C	K	X	M	D	H	X	L	C	N	T	G	C	S
G	L	Y	U	Y	J	J	Y	L	V	N	H	K	U	B	G	S	K	D	Q	D	K	K	L	T	E	C	D	S	P
P	I	F	R	R	M	F	F	L	I	K	B	K	K	J	C	C	I	W	K	J	N	K	E	R	V	C	W	I	H
L	N	M	Y	P	D	T	H	N	T	K	G	M	N	M	N	C	Q	S	Q	B	N	Z	B	B	A	T	L	C	Y
G	J	J	Y	L	Q	N	G	W	J	R	F	G	B	N	Z	I	Y	T	Z	W	Z	B	U	B	R	P	G	I	X
Y	U	D	L	G	Y	I	R	M	L	T	L	Y	T	P	T	T	D	M	M	L	X	T	R	H	T	W	C	X	I
P	R	Y	T	H	T	D	M	C	R	F	K	N	K	V	M	M	Q	A	R	C	R	K	K	G	N	K	K	O	A
K	Y	K	K	I	B	L	W	R	V	X	D	J	R	N	K	T	P	T	E	T	V	H	M	V	I	T	W	P	F
N	V	R	S	L	L	H	B	V	W	K	L	L	C	C	N	G	M	M	Y	H	L	T	K	Z	L	H	R	Y	G
T	N	T	T	M	F	M	Y	X	G	Z	C	L	T	O	X	O	P	L	A	S	M	O	S	I	S	J	X	H	F

20. Epilepsy in Childhood

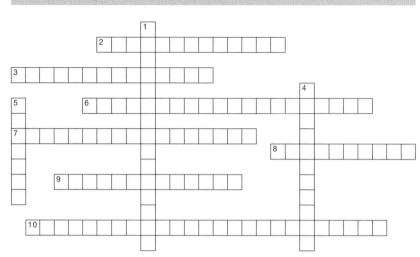

Across

2 Severe epileptic syndrome characterized by different forms of epilepsy, more prevalent in children between the ages of 3 and 5 years (6-7)

3 Common form of epilepsy with the majority never having any further episodes past their teens (6,8)

6 Most useful diagnostic investigation for epilepsy (20)

7 Prolonged or multiple convulsions without recovery of consciousness (6,11)

8 Type of frontal lobe epilepsy (10)

9 Convulsions where consciousness is still intact, originating from a specific area of the brain (6,7)

10 Syndrome consisting of mainly myoclonic seizures, and sometimes absence and tonic–clonic seizures affecting adolescents (8,9,8)

Down

1 From 20 to 30 'salaam' spasms in babies 4–6 months old (9,6)

4 Fit with initial muscle rigidity, then jerk-like movements as well as lack of consciousness (5-6)

5 Staring blankly ahead and loss of consciousness for less than 10 seconds (7)

21. Antiepileptic Drugs

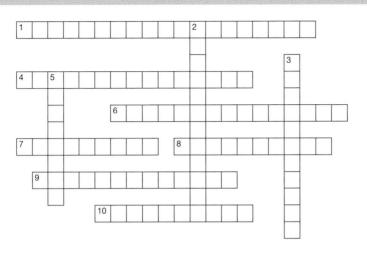

Across

1 Adverse effect of chronic use of phenytoin (8,11)
4 First-line treatment for generalized seizures (6,9)
6 Serious side effect of 9 *Across* that can quickly proceed to death (15)
7 Anticonvulsant associated with toxic effects, such as blood dyscrasia and hirsuitism (9)
8 Drug of choice for infantile spasms (10)
9 First-line treatment for partial seizures (13)
10 Drug with sedative properties particularly effective in the management of myoclonic seizures (10)

Down

2 Antiepileptic used to control absence seizures (12)
3 Second-line treatment for generalized epilepsy known to have few side effects (11)
5 Intravenous administration in status epilepticus (8)

22. Causes of Cough

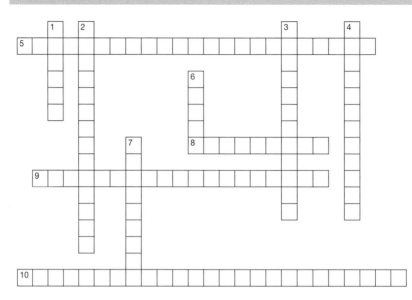

Across

5   A non-respiratory cause of coughing after eating (6-11,6)

8   Coughing spasms with characteristic inspiratory 'whoop' associated with apnoeic episodes followed by vomiting and epitaxis (9)

9   Immotile cilia and dextrocardia (11,8)

10 Organism identified in a wheezy baby 5 months of age with difficulty breathing and intercostal recession (11,9,5)

Down

1   Recurrent cough particularly at night-time and induced by exercise (6)

2   Large quantities of foul-smelling, yellow/green sputum produced (14)

3   Technique to diagnose and remove an aspirated foreign body (12)

4   Persistent cough and a positive Mantoux test (12)

6   Bouts of stridor, barking cough and wheezing mainly during the winter (5)

7   Diagnostic investigation to confirm cystic fibrosis (5,4)

23. Causes of Stridor and Wheeze

Find 18 causes of stridor and wheeze in the grid. Words can go horizontally, vertically and diagonally in all eight directions.

P	X	G	B	N	Y	J	P	R	U	O	M	U	T	L	A	E	G	N	Y	R	A	L
U	U	R	L	R	T	M	L	Y	B	R	T	G	T	V	M	N	W	B	F	K	Z	G
L	L	W	H	T	R	T	S	A	T	R	B	N	F	N	H	G	M	C	W	X	J	N
M	F	D	E	N	A	F	G	Y	R	X	O	N	T	W	W	K	M	M	V	J	T	I
O	E	R	A	T	C	P	C	D	R	Y	L	N	T	J	M	H	N	T	K	N	F	K
N	R	U	R	H	H	L	L	O	K	U	N	Q	C	Z	R	B	X	L	X	F	X	O
A	L	O	T	Y	E	R	B	B	Z	M	E	G	L	H	Q	K	R	G	G	M	P	M
R	A	M	F	R	A	D	M	N	L	H	G	N	O	R	I	K	R	P	F	B	R	S
Y	E	U	A	O	L	M	M	G	T	T	M	T	A	S	B	O	C	M	N	R	T	L
E	G	T	I	T	S	G	F	I	V	K	Q	M	N	C	P	Y	L	L	L	P	D	A
O	A	L	L	O	T	X	C	E	X	M	Y	Y	K	M	I	A	L	I	U	R	D	N
S	H	A	U	X	E	H	P	R	R	C	C	J	T	H	N	T	S	O	T	K	R	R
I	P	N	R	I	N	X	M	O	Q	V	Y	D	G	A	Q	M	R	M	X	I	L	E
N	O	I	E	C	O	M	N	F	D	X	C	Y	P	N	W	C	T	O	K	N	S	T
O	S	T	W	O	S	T	G	T	H	P	Y	H	Z	J	N	Q	W	B	A	T	Q	A
P	E	S	P	S	I	V	X	T	K	D	Y	K	L	Y	T	D	N	R	K	K	C	M
H	O	A	Z	I	S	E	P	I	G	L	O	T	T	I	T	I	S	V	W	A	K	J
I	O	I	J	S	Y	M	Y	N	A	Q	H	L	V	K	G	P	C	K	M	K	Y	D
L	R	D	N	J	K	N	Y	X	T	Y	T	H	H	K	G	Y	H	H	B	X	R	N
I	T	E	N	Q	M	F	I	K	V	X	Q	R	X	T	M	H	T	L	H	D	C	N
A	S	M	J	L	T	S	R	R	Z	H	K	N	T	T	G	S	M	K	R	F	W	D
V	A	S	I	T	I	R	H	T	R	A	D	I	O	T	A	M	U	E	H	R	J	D
T	G	X	J	G	C	T	M	F	C	Y	S	T	I	C	F	I	B	R	O	S	I	S

24. Upper Respiratory Tract Infections

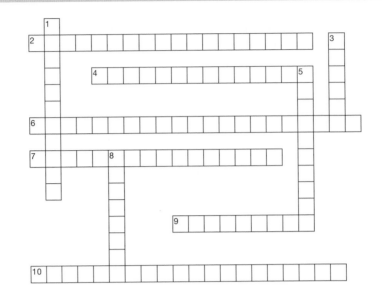

Across

2 Abdominal pain in tonsillitis (10,8)
4 Cardiac complication of streptococcal pharyngitis (9,5)
6 Pathogen responsible for acute epiglottitis (11,10)
7 History of sore throat and running nose (5,11)
9 Facial tenderness and nasal discharge in older children (9)
10 Glue ear (9,6,5)

Down

1 Possible consequence of an inflamed tympanic membrane in otitis media (11)
3 Symptoms of nasal congestion (6)
5 Commonest cause of the common cold (10)
8 Characteristic of exudate indicating a bacterial aetiology of a sore throat (8)

25. Lower Respiratory Tract Infections

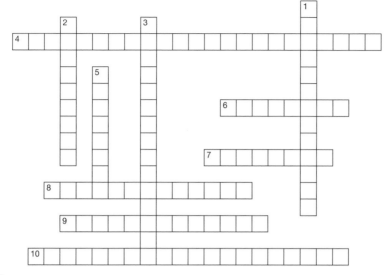

Across

4 Infective agent in lobar pneumonia (13,10)
6 Noisy sound made by babies suggesting respiratory distress (8)
7 Bleeding due to vigorous coughing in whooping cough (8)
8 Dullness on percussion (13)
9 Caused by *Bordetella pertussis* (8,5)
10 Pathogen in schoolchildren with pneumonia (10,10)

Down

1 Wheeze and creptitations in infant <1 year old (13)
2 Neck stiffness only present in some cases of pneumonia (9)
3 Investigation to diagnose *10 Across* (4,11)
5 Individuals most susceptible to group β-haemolytic streptococcus (8)

26. Asthma

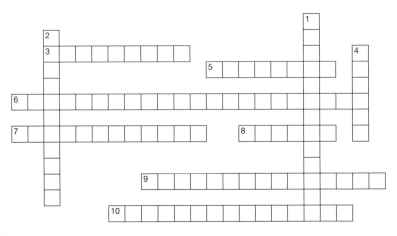

Across

3 Device to administer vaporized medication directly to the lungs (9)
5 Trigger for asthmatic episode (8)
6 Diagnostic investigation in children over 5 years of age (4,10,4,4)
7 Drug given if steroids have had little effect in long-term management (12)
8 Adverse effect of inhaled steroids (6)
9 Symptomatic relief with these drugs (15)
10 Chest deformity suggesting chronic airway obstruction (6,9)

Down

1 Clinical sign of an acute episode found on percussion of the chest (13)
2 Preferred route of administration of aminophylline and hydrocortisone in life-threatening asthma (11)
4 Atopic condition that sometimes coexists with asthma (6)

27. Cystic Fibrosis

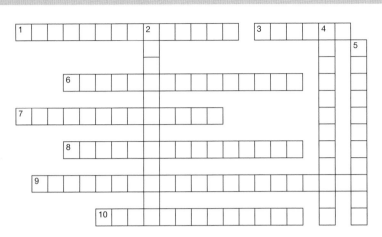

Across

1 Eventual effect of recurrent chest infections (14)
3 Insufficiency of this pancreatic enzyme leads to malabsorption (6)
6 Location of mutant gene (10,5)
7 Intestinal obstruction in neonates (8,5)
8 Obstruction of these leads to malabsorption (10,5)
9 Chronic lung infection caused by a pathogenic species (11,10)
10 Part of disease management (13)

Down

2 CFTR controls its transport (8,4)
4 Gastrointestinal symptom associated with insufficiency of pancreatic enzymes (12)
5 Treatment in the pipeline (4,7)

28. Murmurs

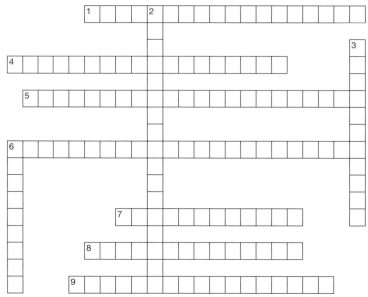

Across

1 Continuous murmur heard at the apex and also at the axilla and back (6,12)

4 Ejection systolic murmur heard at the 3rd intercostal space (6,6,6)

5 Continuous machinery murmur (6,6,10)

6 Pansystolic murmur at the lower left sternal edge (11,6,6)

7 Cause of third heart sound (5,7)

8 Systolic murmur heard at the upper right sternal border which can also be detected in the neck (6,8)

9 Systolic murmur at the upper left sternal edge radiating to the back (9,8)

Down

2 Absent femoral pulse with a systolic ejection murmur heard between the shoulder blades (6,11)

3 Type of murmur which lasts throughout systole (11)

6 Continuous innocent murmur heard below the clavicles (6,3)

29. Clinical Features of Infective Endocarditis

Find 12 clinical features of infective endocarditis in the grid. Words can go horizontally, vertically and diagonally in all eight directions.

Z	Q	J	J	G	B	W	G	W	K	N	B	C	K	E	P	X	R	F	Y
C	P	Y	L	Q	P	F	T	H	N	P	X	N	S	X	R	E	A	L	R
R	X	P	X	G	N	N	R	Q	E	K	K	I	H	T	T	I	G	D	Z
P	U	M	P	V	C	N	X	F	K	A	A	K	M	I	M	F	M	P	K
Q	P	M	P	N	N	Q	V	V	T	L	D	Q	N	E	W	M	S	H	R
N	K	D	R	V	C	H	M	K	A	W	Z	A	A	N	F	R	P	L	L
H	B	N	G	U	C	L	K	M	B	N	L	N	C	K	Q	F	L	M	M
M	D	K	Y	L	M	X	U	G	R	I	A	R	Q	H	P	T	E	C	F
W	W	D	B	L	N	L	G	B	N	L	R	R	R	G	E	K	N	A	C
T	N	M	K	N	B	X	Q	F	B	B	L	P	E	N	T	B	O	I	Q
D	M	P	B	T	D	B	A	G	V	I	V	T	V	T	R	R	M	X	L
H	N	Z	Y	B	Z	R	N	L	N	N	N	R	E	X	R	P	E	E	K
Z	J	K	D	R	C	Y	L	K	M	J	K	G	F	Z	L	N	G	R	G
H	L	M	M	T	B	V	G	F	P	T	Z	P	B	K	P	K	A	O	P
B	N	N	S	Q	Q	F	J	L	Q	M	H	J	F	F	R	Z	L	N	K
R	A	I	G	L	A	R	H	T	R	A	V	F	P	G	Z	C	Y	A	V
S	P	L	I	N	T	E	R	H	A	E	M	O	R	R	H	A	G	E	S
R	N	P	K	H	L	X	D	L	R	W	F	H	H	Y	K	H	L	T	K
Z	Q	Z	M	W	P	W	Y	N	Z	V	T	B	V	Z	F	R	L	R	F
K	R	D	Q	C	E	R	E	B	R	A	L	A	B	S	C	E	S	S	J

30. Congenital Heart Disease

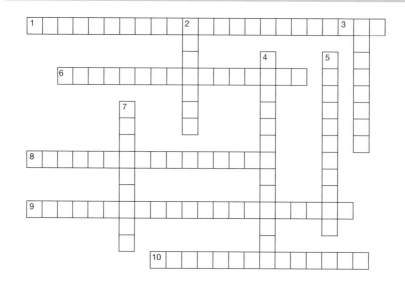

Across

1 Most common congenital heart disease in children (11,6,6)

6 Combination of *1 Across*, right ventricular hypertrophy, pulmonary stenosis and overriding aorta (7,9)

8 Diagnostic investigation that shows most structural cardiac anomalies (16)

9 Antibiotic prophylaxis given before surgery or invasive procedures to prevent this (9,12)

10 Abnormally large opening in atrial septal defect (ASD)(6,8)

Down

2 Maternal disease if acquired during pregnancy can cause heart defects in the fetus (7)

3 Primary symptom of *2 Down* accommodated by the child squatting (8)

4 Congenital disorder associated with ASD (5,8)

5 Typical antibiotic prophylaxis to prevent *9 Across* (11)

7 Drugs taken if heart disease has led to heart failure (9)

31. Anaemia

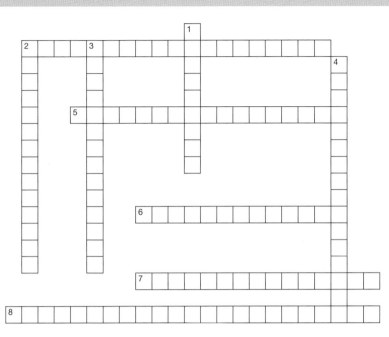

Across

2 Disorder in anaemic teenagers mainly consuming junk food (5,4,10)

5 Afro-Caribbean child presents with anaemia, swollen hands and feet, and a history of repeated episodes of profound pain in long bones and chest (6,4,7)

6 Mild anaemia, jaundice, splenomegaly with an increased risk of gallstones (12)

7 Pancytopenia combined with abnormal radius, hyperpigmentation and high incidence of malignancy (8,7)

8 Blood incompatibility when mothers are Rhesus-negative (6,10,7)

Down

1 Pale skin with bruising, hepatomegaly and lymphadenopathy (9)

2 Prominent forehead present in *4 Down* (7,7)

3 Chronic malabsorption with iron-deficiency anaemia (7,7)

4 A child of Mediterranean descent has severe anaemia, enlarged liver and spleen along with maxillary overgrowth (4,12)

32. Bleeding Disorders

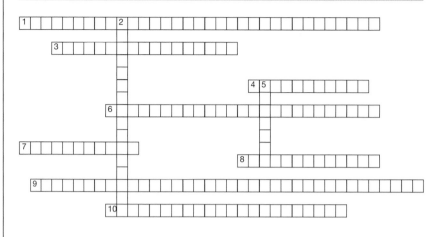

Across

1 Bleeding from mucosal surfaces, for example the mouth and gums (10,16,7)

3 Replacement treatment for 9 *Across* (5,6,6)

4 Deficiency of clotting component in haemophilia A (6,5)

6 Test to see time taken for blood to clot (7,14,4)

7 Male infant presents in first year of life with excessive bleeding (11)

8 Girl presents with easy bruising and epitaxis with a possible family history (3,10)

9 Disorder with features of bleeding from multiple sites as well as blood clots (12,13,11)

10 Presentation of abdominal pain, arthralgia and haemorrhagic rash (6,9,7)

Down

2 Another name for haemophilia B (9,7)

5 Drug that should not be given to patients with bleeding abnormalities (7)

33. Malignancy I

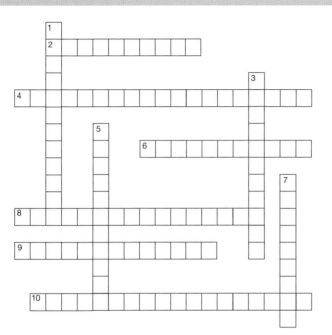

Across

2 Most common site for an astrocytoma to appear (10)

4 Infection to be aware of if a patient is immunocompromised (12,7)

6 Brain tumour which in most cases has a favourable outcome when excised (11)

8 Adolescent with a history of a painless large lump in the neck (8,9)

9 Cells seen on biopsy of *8 Across* (4,9)

10 Commonest form of leukaemia presents in 3–6-year-old children (5,8)

Down

1 Type of leukaemia with a slightly worse prognosis (5,7)

3 'B' symptom of lymphomas (5,6)

5 Chemotherapy to treat ALL (11)

7 Chemotherapeutic agent to treat leukaemia which can have nephrotoxic adverse effects (9)

34. Malignancy II

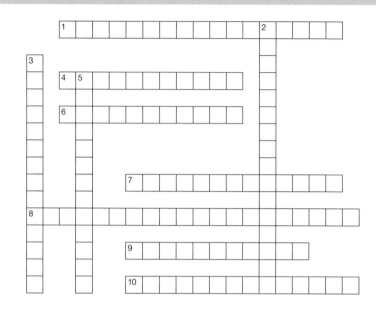

Across

1 An adolescent boy has symptoms of on-going bone pain exacerbated with activity and associated with localized swelling (10,7)

4 Neuroblastoma derived from particular types of cells (6,5)

6 A 3-year-old child presents with large abdominal mass and microscopic haematuria on urinanalysis (5,6)

7 A 2-year-child with an abdominal mass, weight loss and high levels of urinary catecholamines (13)

8 Most common site for benign germ cell tumours (14,6)

9 Treatment offered in advanced cases of nephroblastoma (11)

10 Another name for Wilms' tumour (14)

Down

2 Malignant cause of nasal obstruction with discharge (16)

3 White pupillary reflex detected in neonates (14)

5 Malignancy associated with leg pain, swelling and fracture following a minor fall (6,7)

35. Causes of Tall Stature

Find 14 causes of tall stature in the grid. Words can go horizontally, vertically and diagonally in all eight directions.

B	N	Y	F	R	G	P	M	R	J	N	H	T	G	B	R	F	Q	N	H	B	M	J	N	K	G	F	D
L	R	Y	T	Q	Q	P	R	E	C	O	C	I	O	U	S	P	U	B	E	R	T	Y	N	N	B	D	H
L	M	N	Q	R	R	C	G	F	N	N	H	R	R	F	V	W	M	R	N	L	Z	K	V	T	F	H	G
W	C	X	M	D	K	T	C	N	N	W	N	G	F	K	G	M	P	M	F	L	B	X	J	R	M	T	M
A	I	S	A	L	P	R	E	P	Y	H	L	A	N	E	R	D	A	L	A	T	I	N	E	G	N	O	C
F	C	Y	H	K	K	L	M	T	Z	Y	G	L	M	L	D	D	T	P	M	G	R	L	M	E	G	G	M
T	R	H	M	T	Y	L	Z	T	T	X	R	R	X	K	V	L	X	Y	K	K	M	R	C	M	M	T	V
K	K	D	P	N	F	T	I	I	B	P	C	V	N	B	L	P	N	N	L	R	R	Z	Q	O	M	C	D
C	W	Q	J	N	Q	N	S	N	T	V	T	G	N	N	K	W	T	X	R	Y	R	N	T	R	A	B	C
M	M	C	M	P	C	E	L	M	E	B	X	D	X	R	T	K	H	B	M	K	N	D	M	D	T	T	M
J	S	L	T	X	B	J	Q	M	Y	F	Y	W	H	T	R	K	B	T	N	N	W	W	C	N	E	T	C
M	I	G	Q	O	H	K	K	D	K	H	E	E	R	B	J	K	N	N	P	E	N	V	K	Y	R	K	K
C	D	T	L	N	X	H	D	Q	X	K	Y	L	M	N	G	C	Y	F	M	R	R	P	J	S	N	L	A
F	I	W	Y	X	M	Y	V	N	Q	W	M	V	T	O	A	M	M	O	L	K	K	V	Z	S	A	C	L
H	O	M	O	C	Y	S	T	I	N	U	R	I	A	E	R	C	R	L	L	M	L	L	N	G	L	Q	L
R	R	C	J	W	L	C	W	H	Q	N	G	P	K	B	R	D	R	P	F	F	L	N	K	N	D	B	M
M	Y	T	N	T	L	R	W	Q	K	I	J	C	G	K	N	S	N	O	M	K	W	Z	D	I	I	B	A
Z	H	N	T	P	R	M	C	Y	G	W	L	Y	L	Y	D	C	S	Y	M	L	W	V	P	H	A	W	N
N	T	M	M	F	M	M	W	A	L	W	F	G	S	X	N	T	R	Y	S	E	G	T	P	S	B	T	N
Y	R	N	M	M	V	P	N	D	B	Y	K	S	G	R	Y	F	N	Q	N	S	G	R	K	U	E	J	S
D	E	K	N	H	R	T	M	K	L	V	N	R	K	Z	M	C	W	P	L	D	O	A	Y	C	T	V	S
M	P	H	M	N	I	G	W	R	G	A	B	L	J	L	R	K	Q	M	W	N	R	T	L	Y	E	M	Y
C	Y	V	W	S	N	K	Z	V	F	C	L	K	T	Y	N	M	Z	K	L	C	T	O	O	Y	S	R	N
H	H	L	M	R	R	K	B	R	K	X	B	R	F	V	X	N	X	R	T	R	Q	T	M	S	Z	Q	D
X	T	H	J	R	C	M	A	P	Z	Z	N	L	Z	V	M	T	P	G	N	D	N	T	D	E	R	X	R
P	V	L	J	Q	R	M	R	J	F	R	K	H	K	M	G	K	J	D	K	X	W	N	Q	V	F	Q	O
T	Q	N	G	Z	Q	J	R	P	T	X	R	D	G	G	T	B	M	T	V	M	T	M	R	C	J	J	M
H	V	B	E	C	K	W	I	T	H	W	I	E	D	E	M	A	N	N	S	Y	N	D	R	O	M	E	E

36. Diabetes Mellitus

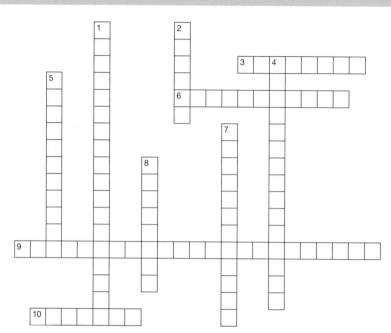

Across

3 Presenting complaint of diabetes (8)

6 Long-term complication suspected in the presence of proteinuria (11)

9 Objective measure of glucose levels in the blood to assess control over the condition (12,13)

10 Products of broken-down fat (7)

Down

1 Preparation given as part of a diabetic regimen (5-6,7)

2 Immediate management in diabetic ketoacidosis to combat dehydration (6)

4 Skin manifestation after repeated injections in the same area of skin (15)

5 Visual complication in diabetes (11)

7 Cause of T-wave changes in diabetic ketoacidosis (12)

8 Deep laboured breathing in metabolic acidosis (8)

37. Causes of Hypoglycaemia

Find 15 causes of hypoglycaemia in the grid. Words can go horizontally, vertically and diagonally in all eight directions.

G	D	W	P	N	D	K	K	H	L	T	W	M	H	T	W	H	M	K	N	P	E	Q	J	T	L	C	M
H	H	T	Z	N	P	J	R	W	K	T	G	Z	T	T	Z	F	W	X	M	S	W	R	I	G	R	O	H
T	R	J	W	J	R	E	C	N	A	C	L	A	N	E	R	D	A	N	A	T	R	N	R	C	P	N	B
W	L	K	M	G	R	B	D	B	T	N	Q	H	P	G	X	Z	G	E	M	C	S	O	N	G	Y	G	J
D	P	A	D	D	I	S	O	N	S	D	I	S	E	A	S	E	S	G	D	U	W	T	K	M	Z	E	P
Y	K	W	R	A	L	C	O	H	O	L	I	S	M	R	H	I	X	W	L	T	H	R	B	L	R	N	M
H	K	L	Q	T	V	Y	K	K	B	K	P	K	R	C	D	R	N	I	H	D	Y	N	R	R	P	I	M
W	Y	J	Z	Q	D	D	M	X	K	J	T	G	F	E	W	T	N	H	M	M	N	A	E	T	T	T	K
K	C	P	R	K	X	H	C	X	F	F	J	H	G	L	P	M	O	T	F	V	G	I	A	K	D	A	F
M	C	D	O	X	C	J	N	Q	J	C	W	A	N	E	N	R	X	L	Y	P	Q	M	S	D	P	L	C
L	T	W	K	P	X	T	M	H	M	C	R	Y	M	M	M	L	J	K	D	Z	K	E	T	Z	G	A	H
M	I	W	P	N	I	M	W	N	N	O	A	O	K	O	S	V	L	G	R	D	R	A	C	Y	M	D	K
T	M	V	C	Q	R	T	R	V	T	K	R	E	N	M	U	H	L	H	Z	K	Z	S	A	K	R	R	V
K	K	Y	E	V	T	R	U	S	R	D	T	E	R	Y	T	M	N	B	N	Y	Y	O	N	H	B	E	F
C	F	D	C	R	W	R	N	I	N	P	D	R	F	U	I	C	D	Q	H	L	C	T	C	L	N	N	N
W	K	N	G	T	D	E	N	Y	T	E	Y	C	T	P	L	L	M	P	K	K	Z	C	E	P	R	A	K
T	K	X	C	N	G	I	S	T	F	A	J	K	Z	Y	L	Y	Y	N	R	T	G	A	R	Y	B	L	C
Q	W	L	N	O	Z	S	S	I	K	N	R	K	N	R	E	D	N	K	Q	H	P	L	Z	H	K	H	R
Q	M	T	C	C	E	N	C	E	C	Z	T	I	F	W	M	X	G	O	P	K	Z	A	X	P	Y	Y	L
C	B	Y	F	Y	H	I	T	L	A	M	W	Z	S	Y	S	M	C	Z	H	H	F	G	Z	M	T	P	Y
P	L	Z	E	T	E	T	N	R	N	S	L	B	T	M	E	H	R	B	T	P	N	K	L	Y	J	E	F
G	Q	R	M	N	J	W	B	K	R	H	E	M	K	P	T	R	T	T	K	J	L	D	K	X	B	R	Q
Q	N	K	C	A	M	O	N	I	L	U	S	N	I	R	E	P	Y	H	P	K	X	U	D	M	K	P	Q
Z	G	Y	L	Y	Q	J	K	L	Y	N	F	N	C	K	B	Q	D	X	F	T	N	T	S	L	M	L	W
Y	T	M	L	Z	W	Z	L	X	L	V	M	K	T	T	A	H	L	Y	R	K	V	N	M	W	J	A	H
F	V	F	T	V	K	N	V	K	T	M	N	K	T	M	I	L	W	P	J	Q	X	F	J	L	H	S	J
Z	K	F	M	R	F	R	Z	K	K	T	Q	Z	T	V	D	M	C	G	T	H	C	M	L	P	K	I	R
L	R	K	T	K	Q	T	X	K	J	M	T	H	K	Z	L	D	P	L	L	Q	M	Q	L	X	P	A	F

38. Endocrine and Metabolic Disorders

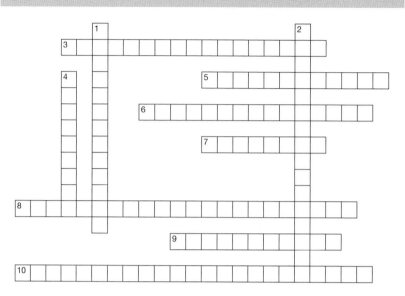

Across

3 Disorder of the pituitary gland with symptoms of thirst and polyuria (8,9)

5 Striking clinical sign seen in adults with hyperthyroidism but uncommon in children (12)

6 Disorder detected by neonatal screening when performing the Guthrie test (15)

7 Inherited disease typically with skin and eye depigmentation (8)

8 Underactive thyroid disease more likely to be found in diabetics and Down's syndrome (8,14)

9 Predominant drug therapy for hyperthyroidism (11)

10 Group of disorders that may cause cardiomyopathy, hepatomegaly, failure to thrive and hypoglycaemia (8,7,8)

Down

1 Neonate cannot metabolize milk products, and develops jaundice, chronic liver disease and cataracts if not treated (13)

2 Can result from chronic corticosteroid usage (8,8)

4 Replacement therapy in hypothyroidism (9)

39. Causes of Neck Lumps

Find 17 causes of lumps in the neck in the grid. Words can go horizontally, vertically and diagonally in all eight directions.

R	D	Y	Z	A	M	O	P	I	L	T	C	V	W	R	K	C	H	K	P	B	F	N	N	L	T	G	V	Y	R
V	Q	T	L	W	T	L	Y	T	T	N	R	R	R	R	K	N	X	C	M	Y	M	P	N	N	H	N	Y	R	M
M	R	P	L	G	L	K	L	L	K	N	Y	P	P	T	R	N	M	L	P	M	C	T	T	N	F	T	Q	T	G
U	P	P	E	R	R	E	S	P	I	R	A	T	O	R	Y	T	R	A	C	T	I	N	F	E	C	T	I	O	N
B	T	P	G	K	X	M	Q	R	T	Z	S	I	S	O	L	U	C	R	E	B	U	T	P	K	L	T	X	R	Q
T	G	C	N	I	N	F	E	C	T	I	O	U	S	M	O	N	O	N	U	C	L	E	O	S	I	S	V	J	R
K	K	T	X	P	Y	J	Z	V	M	D	K	T	R	T	K	T	G	M	R	G	L	Z	L	D	Z	R	L	T	K
K	N	N	K	M	F	R	W	M	L	E	M	D	L	D	Q	A	L	D	Y	F	H	Y	P	M	W	L	G	N	V
M	T	T	T	C	P	X	N	Q	K	R	G	T	R	H	Z	N	M	H	C	R	V	C	M	N	X	Y	L	M	V
D	S	R	N	Y	R	F	H	X	Q	M	M	T	D	V	K	D	K	O	H	W	J	X	L	L	T	R	D	J	L
T	Y	R	W	P	L	N	H	H	X	O	L	F	N	P	V	F	B	L	R	G	D	T	Q	Y	C	C	G	F	K
F	C	U	R	D	V	D	Z	K	G	I	Y	Z	Q	M	J	V	P	G	F	G	R	N	P	W	N	B	M	M	T
D	L	O	M	N	W	X	T	F	K	D	S	Y	H	M	H	K	T	B	K	W	Y	H	K	D	H	P	Z	H	Z
F	A	M	F	P	D	P	X	J	D	C	I	Q	L	L	N	Y	N	S	C	G	D	H	L	L	K	L	Y	T	T
K	I	U	H	H	T	L	D	M	K	Y	T	R	R	C	M	Y	P	X	H	G	C	M	C	L	R	R	B	N	V
H	H	T	T	M	Y	H	N	V	N	S	I	N	B	K	W	M	L	D	K	N	V	D	E	I	O	D	M	R	C
F	C	D	G	A	N	Z	Y	F	T	T	N	R	R	K	U	P	Z	C	T	D	G	U	R	I	T	S	R	M	P
M	N	I	M	S	D	K	L	R	J	M	E	Q	H	M	F	N	T	R	T	H	K	R	D	X	I	S	K	X	C
C	A	O	K	T	R	L	Y	M	O	C	D	B	H	H	M	T	N	F	B	A	Y	C	F	L	D	M	Y	T	T
L	R	T	N	O	R	K	V	T	J	G	A	G	L	K	T	K	H	Q	E	K	A	R	L	L	W	M	Z	C	Z
T	B	S	Z	I	K	P	L	Y	V	G	L	V	Z	B	C	K	V	M	C	R	A	O	O	P	H	X	Y	K	L
M	K	A	N	D	H	N	T	J	C	G	A	O	F	D	C	H	I	W	C	G	C	M	G	I	F	V	V	K	L
R	L	M	N	I	X	K	G	P	K	P	C	G	S	L	F	A	Y	I	R	I	H	L	O	R	D	N	D	M	P
B	N	O	V	T	R	T	T	G	R	G	I	K	H	S	C	B	N	Y	T	W	P	V	J	H	V	I	H	C	X
J	G	N	N	I	Q	T	F	Q	L	G	V	B	R	M	A	O	L	R	L	F	H	G	H	Q	P	B	T	W	T
F	T	R	N	S	L	D	B	M	V	N	R	W	Q	R	M	L	O	F	M	N	T	H	J	L	X	M	D	I	J
L	F	E	T	K	N	Z	Z	Z	G	L	E	M	W	A	J	T	C	K	N	P	G	F	L	T	L	K	Y	H	S
J	Z	T	X	R	D	P	R	T	J	N	C	M	R	X	P	M	C	Y	X	L	X	N	K	M	L	M	R	L	N
J	Y	S	L	B	N	G	C	N	G	M	W	T	D	L	K	N	Z	N	S	X	T	N	P	K	C	C	K	K	P
K	J	P	N	L	L	Q	T	F	K	V	N	Y	D	P	J	J	J	V	X	V	T	K	B	M	R	W	T	F	R	F

40. Leg Pain and Limp

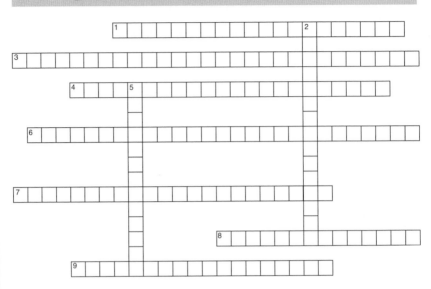

Across

1 Most common pathogen causing *5 Down* (14,6)
3 Adolescent overweight boy with a limp combined with hip and knee pain (7,5,7,9)
4 Sporty adolescent boy presents with pain below the patella that worsens with exercise (6-9)
6 Used to be called Still's disease (8,10,9)
7 Hip dislocated out of acetabulum in neonates (13,9)
8 Pain in hip, leg or knee confirmed on x-ray of a 'flattened' femoral head (7,7)
9 Afebrile child limping with hip pain following an upper respiratory tract infection (9,9)

Down

2 Unwell child holding a limb with a warm, tender joint (6,9)
5 Following an injury, fever with severe bone pain and joint swelling (13)

41. Disorders of the Back

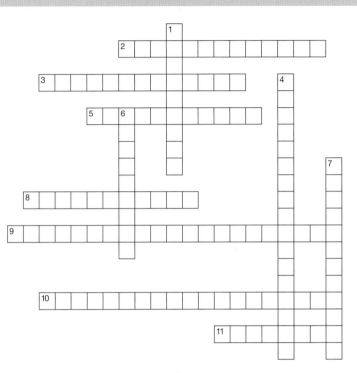

Across

2 Stress fracture in the lower back of adolescent athletes (13)

3 Systemically unwell young child with localized pain and swelling (13)

5 Caused by repetitive strain or trauma from a sports-related injury (6,5)

8 A wry neck (11)

9 A 15-year-old with back pain, worse in the morning yet improves throughout the day (10,11)

10 Round-back deformity of the thoracic spine most common in adolescents (12,7)

11 Disc space infection typically presenting as severe back pain with insidious onset (8)

Down

1 Main form of treatment for back pain, especially if it is muscular in origin (9)

4 In cases of 2 Across where the vertebra shifts backwards (17)

6 Painless lateral curvature deformity of the spine in adolescents (9)

7 Back pain in a child diagnosed with tuberculosis (5,7)

42. Acute Rashes I

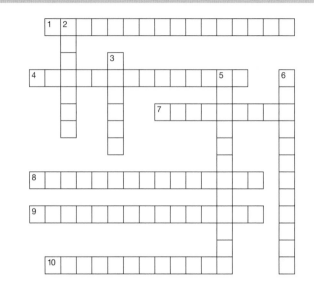

Across

1 Relatively common complication of measles (16)

4 Cardiac complication of *6 Down* occurring very rarely in developed countries (9,5)

7 Itchy rash with characteristic weals surrounded by erythematous skin (9)

8 Uncommon rash more prevalent in Japanese children with a complication of coronary aneurysms (8,7)

9 Intravenous treatment to prevent coronary complications in *8 Across* (15)

10 Clinical sign of measles seen in the mouth during the prodromal phase (7,5)

Down

2 Mild rash during childhood, but if acquired during pregnancy can have serious consequences on fetal development (7)

3 Red, circumscribed flat lesion that blanches on pressure (6)

5 Uncommon but serious complication of measles (12)

6 Cause of maculopapular rash with 'white strawberry' tongue (7,5)

43. Acute Rashes II

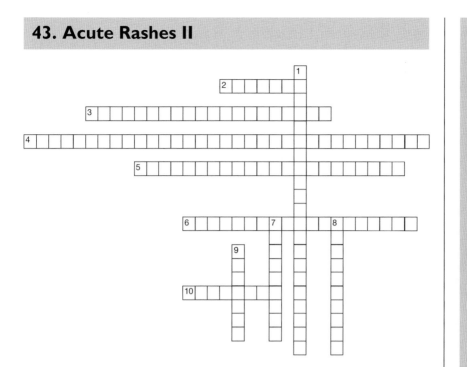

Across

2　Serum-filled, raised lesion (<5 mm diameter), e.g. present in chickenpox (7)

3　Pearly white wart-like lesion on skin (9,11)

4　Acute onset of purpura and bruising on the skin as well as bleeding from the gums and nose (10,16,7)

5　Childhood disorder with features of a symmetrical purpuric rash on buttocks and limbs, in combination with arthritis and abdominal pain (6-9,7)

6　Maculopapular 'lace-like' rash on arms, thighs and trunk with the 'slapped cheek' appearance (8,11)

10　Vesicle with honey-coloured exudate on the face (8)

Down

1　Infective agent that should be suspected in a febrile child with a purpuric rash (9,12)

7　Treatment given to the immunocompromised if they acquire chickenpox (9)

8　Generalized, intensely itchy, macular rash which progresses to papules, then to vesicles, and lastly to pustules with crusting (10)

9　Raised lesion with clear or purulent fluid (7)

44. Causes of Purpuric Rashes

Find 19 causes of purpuric rashes in the grid. Words can go horizontally, vertically and diagonally in all eight directions.

L	M	K	G	H	A	F	F	J	B	Z	X	Y	P	O	S	T	T	R	A	N	S	F	U	S	I	O	N	H	N	K	L	Z	L	C	P
T	D	H	J	N	R	W	F	R	J	L	J	T	P	N	N	Y	N	G	Z	B	R	L	D	N	L	R	J	T	O	C	K	K	B	R	F
L	X	Q	T	J	U	P	N	D	C	J	V	R	V	T	T	R	J	R	H	C	F	R	V	K	T	P	P	L	I	L	J	X	Y	H	V
R	M	J	P	R	P	Y	F	M	Q	M	C	L	L	B	T	R	R	B	M	R	Q	R	B	T	W	M	R	V	T	Y	N	G	B	K	M
T	R	W	Q	C	R	N	F	Q	L	K	H	T	Q	V	X	C	X	Q	D	T	M	L	P	M	N	H	E	T	A	C	W	T	R	N	D
M	T	W	A	R	U	P	R	U	P	N	I	E	L	N	O	H	C	S	H	C	O	N	E	H	V	N	Y	S	L	N	F	L	R	X	R
Q	M	N	Z	L	P	K	G	C	V	L	B	N	N	N	T	W	B	N	Y	F	L	M	R	T	I	Y	T	H	U	L	R	M	N	V	K
K	H	K	J	M	C	T	R	L	E	U	K	A	E	M	I	A	G	D	Z	W	K	H	C	N	V	E	B	T	G	F	Z	X	Q	W	C
T	P	T	J	F	I	Z	R	F	G	R	J	Q	M	N	W	K	K	F	J	D	J	L	I	K	R	H	X	Z	A	B	F	M	P	T	F
T	N	N	B	B	N	R	A	R	L	L	G	B	L	N	Y	G	M	F	G	L	M	U	Q	O	Y	T	H	Q	O	V	W	T	L	F	R
K	R	T	Z	K	E	F	T	I	B	Y	C	B	N	F	G	N	N	K	W	C	Q	Y	I	X	K	Z	S	F	C	L	N	L	X	K	T
H	C	Y	T	T	P	R	K	Z	M	M	F	N	B	B	N	T	K	R	P	W	C	D	G	F	X	U	K	Y	R	R	R	V	L	V	R
C	M	N	Z	M	O	Y	K	R	C	E	C	V	B	C	G	K	W	N	V	K	S	D	C	Q	S	L	N	R	A	V	C	F	W	N	K
M	X	K	M	P	T	H	X	C	B	K	A	H	A	J	T	G	V	M	K	D	L	M	J	O	Q	X	X	R	L	V	Y	X	D	Z	H
T	Q	M	N	B	C	G	L	L	F	N	C	C	L	P	X	W	P	Y	C	L	W	D	T	V	L	Z	F	M	U	R	L	T	R	N	O
K	R	Q	L	T	O	M	R	L	L	M	K	C	I	P	L	M	F	Z	G	Y	H	A	Z	D	D	W	M	X	C	G	L	K	N	Y	S
Q	K	R	T	T	B	N	K	V	R	L	V	M	Z	T	R	A	Q	R	Q	W	M	G	D	G	B	K	E	R	S	M	G	Q	K	T	T
N	L	P	C	M	M	J	T	M	T	K	L	F	T	X	P	R	S	K	D	E	M	F	L	L	K	H	T	Z	A	Q	N	X	T	Y	E
I	F	B	N	G	O	D	N	D	K	G	J	M	M	C	T	E	N	T	H	H	F	P	M	N	L	W	Q	M	V	K	N	M	W	T	O
C	N	B	Q	L	R	W	B	M	C	R	K	V	Y	P	I	K	S	T	I	M	P	R	P	E	W	P	B	H	A	L	T	L	T	T	G
I	P	Z	J	T	H	A	V	T	N	J	R	F	X	R	L	H	Y	L	P	C	N	N	R	X	N	Z	K	R	R	T	D	D	K	P	E
P	Q	R	N	X	T	M	H	R	L	L	M	K	N	B	P	R	T	T	A	P	A	S	M	T	N	B	J	X	T	N	L	Q	L	K	N
M	R	R	C	G	C	Y	Y	W	W	B	L	A	K	K	E	M	D	A	K	C	D	N	M	R	K	N	B	Q	N	Q	L	J	K	L	E
A	Y	Y	Y	V	I	L	T	B	N	T	R	J	R	S	K	K	Z	D	P	A	C	Q	A	T	T	N	L	B	I	T	J	W	P	Z	S
F	Q	M	N	M	H	O	L	M	H	R	T	B	U	F	Y	K	Y	M	N	O	W	O	T	E	M	H	A	R	D	N	V	L	P	J	I
I	L	X	W	G	T	I	X	V	G	K	G	P	X	B	A	H	J	L	R	K	I	X	C	H	M	I	V	L	E	K	R	Z	K	L	S
R	K	K	K	C	A	D	K	F	L	P	U	K	X	K	W	N	O	Q	M	Q	T	D	G	O	R	I	L	V	T	N	G	H	H	R	I
Y	R	P	Y	Z	P	Z	Z	D	Z	L	R	P	G	R	Y	S	S	C	M	F	M	M	I	E	G	T	A	K	A	N	Z	C	N	V	M
F	T	K	J	M	O	F	W	C	C	V	G	W	Y	G	S	T	Q	S	K	M	L	C	H	G	J	N	P	V	N	M	J	N	V	G	P
R	R	R	K	H	I	N	J	I	T	L	Y	T	K	Y	X	Z	Q	L	Y	Y	H	T	N	M	N	B	I	Z	I	M	J	T	K	C	E
T	W	M	M	R	D	K	M	K	L	Z	Q	Y	N	L	D	L	C	L	W	N	H	T	F	J	Q	K	W	N	M	N	V	M	G	V	R
D	N	T	B	V	I	E	X	K	G	J	X	D	M	L	X	D	B	T	J	P	D	Y	W	P	X	Q	H	K	E	W	T	R	F	N	F
D	F	L	C	J	T	V	M	M	D	F	R	X	F	K	Z	X	M	K	I	T	M	R	C	H	M	Q	R	K	S	M	C	T	F	T	E
L	C	B	T	S	F	N	N	M	T	O	B	B	R	J	C	L	L	D	P	R	W	C	O	L	N	X	X	N	S	J	W	G	P	X	C
F	J	F	Y	N	V	T	K	Y	M	G	G	B	C	I	N	E	G	O	H	C	Y	S	P	M	M	H	N	C	I	N	K	N	K	R	T
B	Y	S	V	A	R	I	C	E	L	L	A	Z	O	S	T	E	R	K	C	M	T	V	J	Q	E	J	H	M	D	M	R	R	M	W	A

45. Management of Chronic Skin Disorders

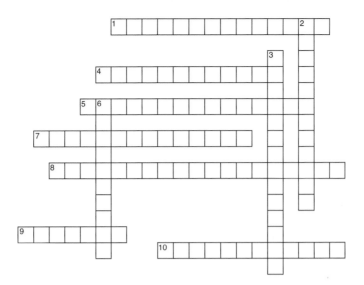

Across

1 Ointment to remove psoriatic plaques (10,4)
4 Oral antibiotic for pustular acne (12)
5 Topical bacteriocidal medication causing skin peeling in the treatment of acne (7,8)
7 Apply to affected area during acute exacerbations of eczema (14)
8 First-line treatment for plaque psoriasis (4,3,12)
9 Form of psoriasis more common in children (7)
10 Alternative to drug therapy in the management of eczema, psoriasis and acne (12)

Down

2 Treatment of choice for severe pustular acne vulgaris (12)
3 Drugs to relieve itching in eczema (14)
4 Preparations to moisturize the skin in atopic eczema (10)

46. Causes of Acute Fever

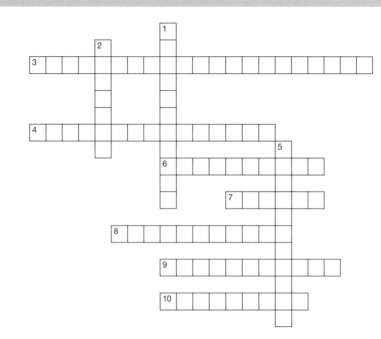

Across

3 Fever accompanied by symptoms of frequency, dysuria and enuresis (7,5,9)

4 Joint inflammation and pain accompanying a fever and chills (6,9)

6 Child presents with fever, headache and vomiting (10)

7 Method of taking core body temperature (6)

8 Fever associated with sore throat and on examination white exudate seen on the tonsils (11)

9 Microorganisms in the blood that is often asymptomatic (11)

10 Dry cough, tachypnoea and pyrexia caused by a virus (9)

Down

1 An antipyretic (11)

2 Fever after international travel (7)

5 High fever with red, bulging eardrum on examination (6,5)

47. Causes of Pyrexia of Unknown Origin

Find 15 causes of pyrexia of an unknown origin in the grid. Words can go horizontally, vertically and diagonally in all eight directions.

B	B	K	R	L	L	L	K	K	N	M	S	G	B	G	R	A	K	N	L	S	R	P	A	F	K
L	L	W	N	R	W	R	R	V	Q	I	G	P	K	L	I	K	Q	K	L	Y	T	G	I	I	N
M	M	W	R	N	N	F	W	X	S	L	W	D	N	N	Y	R	R	R	S	M	R	M	N	I
H	Q	N	H	R	B	N	R	O	F	T	Q	C	O	T	R	K	V	I	H	T	C	N	E	F	N
T	M	H	M	N	H	V	L	T	F	R	T	M	I	D	W	Y	C	G	Z	E	L	M	A	L	F
L	B	P	P	D	B	L	T	R	H	N	U	K	T	Q	M	W	N	X	K	M	C	E	K	A	E
M	N	N	V	N	E	V	F	C	G	E	F	G	C	R	H	T	H	R	C	I	M	D	U	M	C
J	V	N	F	C	M	N	V	T	N	V	R	L	E	L	L	L	B	V	G	C	R	I	E	M	T
W	J	F	U	M	Z	W	P	P	U	R	P	G	F	Y	B	M	T	L	N	L	W	T	L	A	I
L	C	R	T	N	M	N	M	Y	P	B	J	M	N	L	Q	W	B	R	C	U	N	E	N	T	O
R	B	F	R	V	X	Q	M	X	Q	M	E	W	I	K	D	F	C	M	Y	P	P	R	M	O	U
L	Y	M	P	H	O	M	A	T	D	J	R	R	T	Q	B	C	G	G	M	U	V	R	K	R	S
I	N	F	E	C	T	I	V	E	E	N	D	O	C	A	R	D	I	T	I	S	M	A	T	Y	M
T	P	X	R	J	G	Z	F	B	F	T	B	Y	A	U	Z	K	B	H	L	E	O	N	P	B	O
T	K	T	M	R	D	L	M	C	D	T	J	V	R	K	L	H	Y	W	H	R	S	E	J	O	N
J	G	C	Q	G	P	G	H	P	T	D	G	Q	T	P	K	O	N	T	H	Y	T	A	M	W	O
M	X	T	L	K	L	H	M	L	H	N	L	L	Y	T	G	C	S	T	N	T	E	N	G	E	N
J	L	Q	L	X	M	V	J	L	J	H	H	L	R	M	Q	M	Q	I	R	H	O	F	K	L	U
K	X	X	K	M	A	K	Y	N	T	E	R	G	A	G	K	Y	B	W	S	E	M	E	C	D	C
M	V	F	B	Z	R	I	B	C	P	X	M	R	N	D	J	B	V	H	T	M	Y	V	W	I	L
M	F	L	Y	Q	F	D	R	A	K	B	R	F	I	K	T	C	K	N	K	A	E	E	L	S	E
L	P	M	V	N	V	G	T	A	G	F	L	B	R	M	C	B	R	L	V	T	L	R	R	E	O
D	R	V	J	D	B	I	C	N	L	G	H	K	U	H	V	G	M	H	B	O	I	D	F	A	S
X	R	M	K	N	T	D	G	N	A	L	J	Y	L	Z	V	F	T	Q	S	T	P	B	S	I
J	K	R	N	I	V	P	Z	K	K	V	M	N	K	R	K	N	Y	F	W	U	I	L	W	E	S
L	Y	G	S	X	K	R	W	Q	F	X	R	L	Z	D	M	L	L	M	N	S	S	T	B	L	N

48. Shock

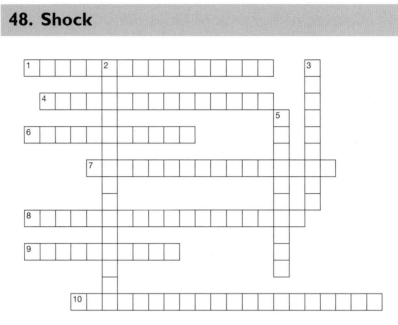

Across

1 Drug that should be administered if *7 Across* is suspected (16)

4 Hypovolaemic shock caused by loss of bodily fluids (15)

6 Early stage of shock in which the vital organs are still perfused (11)

7 Child presents with manifestations of septicaemic shock combined with purpuric rash and neck stiffness (16)

8 Quick access to circulation if you are struggling to attain intravenous access (12,6)

9 Effective means of delivering oxygen to a child in an emergency situation (3,3,4)

10 Cause of shock in cases of consistently high glucose levels (8,12)

Down

2 Result of anaphylactic shock causing hoarseness and stridor (9,6)

3 Electrolyte added to saline in the management of *10 Across* (9)

5 Intramuscular injection for immediate management of anaphylactic shock (10)

49. Causes of a Coma

Find 15 causes of a coma in the grid. Words can go horizontally, vertically and diagonally in all eight directions.

G	D	C	S	U	C	I	T	P	E	L	I	P	E	S	U	T	A	T	S
X	G	L	N	M	Q	W	N	T	T	K	N	B	L	L	Y	M	K	T	M
S	I	S	O	D	I	C	A	O	T	E	K	C	I	T	E	B	A	I	D
C	L	H	T	B	L	Y	Q	M	B	M	S	M	Y	Q	E	B	D	K	M
A	J	F	H	G	F	P	S	Y	M	I	H	H	R	G	M	I	C	R	P
R	R	K	W	Y	H	W	Z	T	T	K	Y	V	N	M	O	R	F	Y	L
D	N	L	J	H	P	K	V	I	R	P	T	I	C	L	R	T	W	R	C
I	K	K	Z	T	T	O	G	L	O	O	N	W	B	V	D	H	T	U	T
A	F	T	R	D	T	N	N	G	R	O	K	J	X	F	N	A	K	J	Y
C	J	L	T	Y	I	R	L	A	S	H	L	E	L	T	Y	S	L	N	L
A	R	Z	L	N	N	Y	Z	I	T	M	R	M	R	D	S	P	L	I	M
R	I	K	E	J	C	N	O	T	K	R	J	G	P	N	S	H	F	D	J
R	T	M	Z	A	N	P	T	D	G	V	A	W	W	L	E	Y	B	A	J
E	J	T	E	N	D	N	Q	C	L	G	K	E	R	L	Y	X	Z	E	Z
S	N	M	N	A	W	Y	L	X	Z	F	C	F	M	X	E	I	J	H	N
T	I	R	E	N	R	N	R	G	K	R	K	K	J	I	R	A	N	F	N
A	M	L	R	M	G	U	L	V	Z	T	K	N	X	R	A	L	F	H	V
M	M	K	W	N	G	L	K	E	N	C	E	P	H	A	L	I	T	I	S
T	R	U	O	M	U	T	L	A	I	N	A	R	C	A	R	T	N	I	N
N	G	B	K	H	Y	D	R	O	C	E	P	H	A	L	U	S	P	Q	W

50. Poisoning

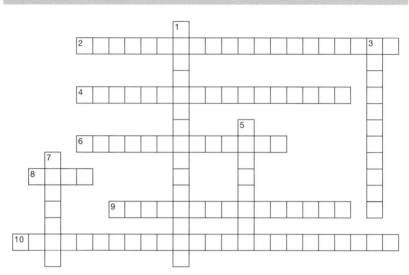

Across

2 Overdose of aspirin causes this (11,9)
4 Preparation used to adsorb some drugs (9,8)
6 Technique performed in cases of large overdose or unconscious patient (7,6)
8 Substance given in bleach poisoning (4)
9 Chelating agent used in iron poisoning (15)
10 Child presents with cardiac arrhythmia, drowsiness and blurred vision after ingesting this type of medication (9,15)

Down

1 Treatment given in paracetamol poisoning (1-14)
3 Syrup to induce vomiting (11)
5 Antidote for excessive opiate ingestion (8)
7 Overdose of cardiac drug results in arrhythmia and high potassium levels (7)

51. Non-Accidental Injury

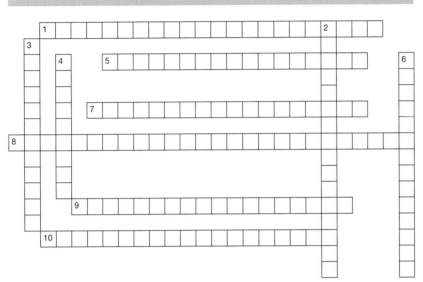

Across

1 Disorder with features of recurrent fractures, blue sclera and deafness at an early age that can be mistaken for abuse (12,10)

5 Syndrome in which a child is hospitalized with a fabricated illness (10,2,5)

7 A battered child with long-term neurological injury (5,4,8)

8 Head injury unlikely to be caused by a fall (9,9,8)

9 Typical physical feature of abuse, particularly if the baby is shaken (7,11)

10 Most common intracranial lesion associated with child abuse (8,11)

Down

2 Child not provided with adequate support, love and affection (9,7)

3 A consequence of facial blows (4,8)

4 Ribs crushed from chest compression (9)

6 Circular, clearly-defined blisters with erythematous edges (8,5)

52. Child Immunizations

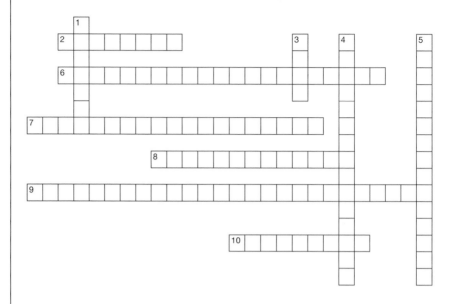

Across

2 To determine whether a child has been exposed to tuberculosis (4,4)
6 Tuberculosis vaccine (7,8-6)
7 Triple vaccine given to infants 12–15 months old (7,5,7)
8 Live, attenuated vaccine (13)
9 Immunization against epiglottitis and the main cause of meningitis in young children (11,10,4,1)
10 Part of triple therapy given at 2, 3 and 4 months of age (9)

Down

1 Booster given if an individual has had wound contamination and not been immunized (7)
3 7 *Across* should not given to children if there is a history of anaphylaxis to these (4)
4 Should not receive live vaccines if on this medication (15)
5 Administered to neonates whose mothers have chickenpox (15)

53. Maternal Conditions and Drugs Affecting Fetal Development

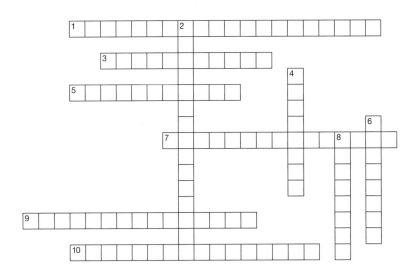

Across

1 Risk to fetus when excessive alcohol is consumed (5,7,8)
3 Complication of drug abuse in pregnancy (11)
5 Devastating teratogenic drug prevalent in the 1960s (11)
7 Congenital viral infection, acquired from the mother, responsible for cataracts, learning disabilities and scarring of the skin in an infant (9,6)
9 Antiepileptic drug related to increased risk of neural tube defects (6,9)
10 Parasite passed on through contact with infected cat faeces (10,6)

Down

2 Most common infection acquired transparentally (15)
4 Anticoagulant that should not be given during the first trimester of pregnancy (8)
6 Complication of the rubella infection (8)
8 Intrauterine infection that can be treated with parenteral penicillin (8)

54. Birth Injuries and Asphyxia

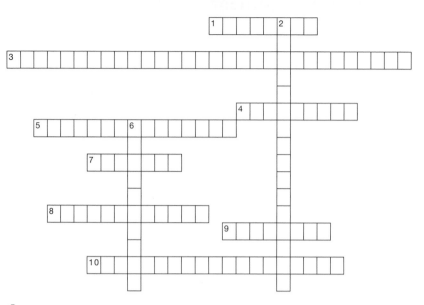

Across

1 Bone most likely to be fractured during birth (8)

3 Brain injury in an asphyxiated infant (7,9,14)

4 Injury affecting the upper brachial plexus (4,5)

5 Bruising on the head of a baby due to instrumental delivery or prolonged stage II of labour (15)

7 Temporary oedema following a ventose delivery (7)

8 Nerve palsy weakening the muscles of the wrist and fingers (7,5)

9 Substance passed by the fetus during labour or birth, which could indicate fetal distress (8)

10 Mass in the infant's neck due to bleeding and trauma (13,6)

Down

2 Swelling of the scalp caused by mechanical trauma during delivery, resolving in days (5,11)

6 Quantitative method to evaluate a baby's physical condition 1 and 5 minutes after birth (5,5)

55. Complications of Preterm Babies

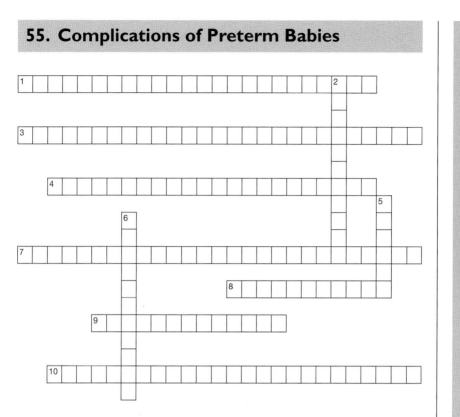

Across

1 Gastrointestinal emergency more common in preterm infants (13,11)
3 Lesions that can be seen on cranial ultrasounds (16,11)
4 Cardiac complication associated with RDS (6,6,10)
7 Serious complication due to pulmonary surfactant deficiency (11,8,8)
8 Poor thermoregulation (11)
9 Metabolic complication (13)
10 Chronic lung disease (16,9)

Down

2 Less than a certain number of weeks for the gestation period for a baby to be considered as premature (6,5)
5 Episodes of cession of breathing (6)
6 Disorder found in premature babies that can lead to blindness (11)

56. Causes of Neonatal Jaundice

Find 19 causes of neonatal jaundice in the grid. Words can go horizontally, vertically and diagonally in all eight directions.

P	Y	R	U	V	A	T	E	K	I	N	A	S	E	D	E	F	I	C	I	E	N	C	Y
D	R	R	X	Q	L	V	X	R	L	B	G	A	L	A	C	T	O	S	A	E	M	I	A
U	G	N	X	N	R	H	D	M	D	L	K	L	T	L	J	H	V	Z	R	N	D	N	M
B	E	S	A	E	S	I	D	S	U	S	E	H	R	T	K	Z	D	E	O	O	E	H	B
I	W	N	F	H	K	F	K	Q	L	P	X	M	N	T	M	K	L	M	T	I	M	L	J
N	P	D	H	Y	N	N	C	K	K	N	D	L	L	X	F	M	Y	O	O	T	O	P	E
J	C	X	K	N	S	I	T	I	G	N	I	N	E	M	X	G	T	R	R	C	R	C	S
O	R	Y	Y	L	F	Q	D	R	W	T	B	G	P	V	R	R	I	D	S	E	D	R	A
H	T	M	S	D	L	B	P	W	G	L	W	F	T	R	M	X	L	N	S	F	N	T	E
N	G	C	W	T	B	I	R	T	H	T	R	A	U	M	A	G	I	Y	Y	N	Y	J	S
S	G	Y	P	M	I	H	P	T	Z	V	J	X	P	X	X	A	B	S	N	I	S	M	I
O	P	T	Q	T	L	C	D	S	B	T	V	C	Z	M	I	B	I	S	D	T	R	H	D
N	R	O	R	D	T	G	F	V	P	R	H	H	M	S	H	N	T	T	R	C	A	Z	L
S	T	M	M	M	Y	R	M	I	W	H	E	L	E	K	L	C	A	R	O	A	J	L	L
Y	F	E	R	Z	L	K	T	Y	B	P	E	R	F	M	V	L	P	E	M	R	J	Q	E
N	J	G	L	A	T	W	R	R	A	R	T	R	T	T	L	Z	M	B	E	T	A	X	C
D	Y	A	B	D	I	W	B	T	M	A	O	L	O	E	K	C	O	L	K	Y	N	Y	E
R	H	L	Y	P	H	N	I	L	Y	D	H	S	B	C	N	Q	C	I	N	R	R	R	L
O	M	O	M	L	M	T	O	R	R	F	R	U	I	T	Y	M	N	G	K	A	E	C	K
M	B	V	R	R	I	R	A	M	M	W	R	Y	L	S	N	T	I	C	T	N	L	Z	C
E	Y	I	V	S	B	I	C	P	U	L	W	J	N	L	X	K	O	L	M	I	G	Q	I
N	T	R	B	K	L	L	C	M	L	E	T	T	G	G	X	C	B	S	V	R	I	X	S
C	J	U	X	I	J	N	T	V	F	R	N	J	J	L	G	M	A	V	I	U	R	V	D
Q	B	S	B	T	M	G	M	Z	B	X	K	P	R	N	X	Z	P	K	K	S	C	J	K

57. Convulsions in Neonates

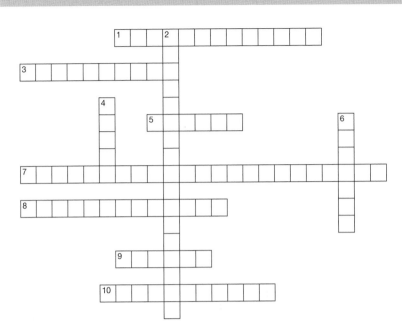

Across

1　A metabolic cause of fits that can be prevented by feeding milk soon after birth (13)

3　Intracranial infection that must always be considered (10)

5　Type of seizure that manifests as prolonged normal activities, e.g. chewing (6)

7　Convulsions more often found in preterm babies (12,11)

8　Electrolyte imbalance cause (13)

9　Convulsions related to rhythmic movements, especially one extremity or one side of the body (6)

10　Similar to seizures but without occular involvement (11)

Down

2　Baby stops breathing due to a blockage in the airways (11,6)

4　Seizure causing stiffening of the limbs or trunk (5)

6　Maternal drug withdrawal causes convulsions in the baby (7)

58. Causes of Neonatal Apnoea

Find 18 causes of neonatal apnoea in the grid. Words can go horizontally, vertically and diagonally in all eight directions.

N	M	K	Y	K	C	K	R	V	M	F	W	T	D	T	R	C	B	B	K	G	V	T	L
E	R	C	D	K	L	K	K	M	R	R	Q	Z	K	N	N	Q	I	P	V	K	X	T	D
C	K	A	I	M	E	A	C	L	A	C	R	E	P	Y	H	N	N	A	P	Z	U	L	F
R	N	P	M	X	G	R	C	D	J	P	K	N	V	G	M	A	T	T	M	F	L	F	V
O	G	J	P	B	M	E	N	I	N	G	I	T	I	S	R	I	R	E	V	G	F	K	Q
T	Z	M	F	P	F	P	R	A	N	A	E	M	I	A	R	M	A	N	L	L	E	T	N
I	T	G	Z	L	N	R	T	Y	M	W	C	K	Y	V	M	E	C	T	F	L	R	M	R
Z	T	K	Q	K	R	E	K	T	D	T	E	R	Q	S	V	A	R	D	H	N	L	K	P
I	B	K	K	H	D	Y	U	K	Z	R	D	N	L	R	G	C	A	U	X	V	A	M	Q
N	G	M	N	Z	R	P	H	M	N	K	M	D	T	E	X	Y	N	C	T	M	E	T	R
G	C	Q	K	G	A	N	D	I	O	J	R	K	T	K	Y	L	I	T	M	J	G	R	P
E	M	O	T	Z	T	I	C	J	Y	N	D	P	W	C	K	G	A	U	H	P	A	A	W
N	N	G	N	D	G	T	M	N	R	C	I	M	G	O	Q	O	L	S	J	Q	H	C	T
T	P	K	W	V	E	Y	N	R	Q	G	A	A	X	L	T	P	H	A	J	Y	P	H	K
E	Y	R	V	R	U	K	Y	C	E	C	C	T	R	B	R	Y	A	R	M	N	O	E	W
R	G	L	U	V	G	L	T	F	R	H	K	D	S	A	T	H	E	T	V	M	S	O	K
O	W	S	D	M	B	J	S	O	R	B	T	E	G	T	K	Y	M	E	K	F	E	M	C
C	J	P	W	H	H	Y	G	I	X	R	V	O	L	E	T	L	O	R	V	L	O	A	Y
O	M	W	W	P	C	L	S	K	O	I	R	R	P	B	D	H	R	I	M	J	O	L	N
L	F	F	C	K	O	I	P	G	T	N	R	Q	W	Y	P	L	R	O	H	R	R	A	B
I	Y	L	K	S	S	V	F	A	L	M	S	B	N	K	H	M	H	S	W	Z	T	C	G
T	M	H	S	P	R	F	D	J	X	T	J	V	L	C	X	T	A	U	W	N	S	I	Q
I	K	I	E	Q	Q	E	D	Q	A	I	X	Y	H	P	S	A	G	S	Y	M	A	A	L
S	A	S	H	C	S	J	L	L	F	J	H	B	F	P	P	R	E	N	M	K	G	Z	H

59. Psychological Disorders in Adolescence

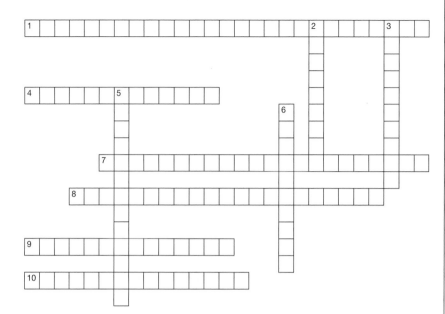

Across

1 Persistent thoughts and repetitive behaviour, common in this age-group (9,10,8)

4 Long-term psychiatric disorder with its initial symptoms appearing in late adolescence (13)

7 Disorder with non-specific signs and symptoms, such as myalgia and poor concentration, occurring post-viral infection (7,7,8)

8 Psychological disorder in which a person tends to act impulsively, inducing acts of violence and self-harm (10,11)

9 Showing signs of frequent vomiting and tendency to binge-eating (7,7)

10 Condition with features of significant weight loss along with a distorted view of their own body image (8,7)

Down

2 Sufferers of 9 Across have been known to take these medications to avoid weight gain (9)

3 Low mood (10)

5 Therapy used to unearth deep-seated conflicts (13)

6 Clinical sign of starvation (6,4)

60. Substance Misuse

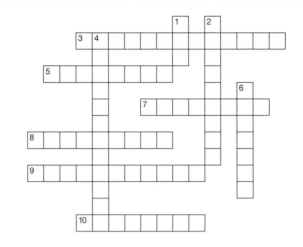

Across

3 LSD, angel dust and magic mushrooms are all part of this group (13)

5 Pupil reaction when taking opiates (8)

7 Recreational drug used for enhancing mood and relaxation (8)

8 Given as a long-term maintenance therapy to heroin addicts (9)

9 Effect of cocaine in which a person feels insects are crawling under their skin (11)

10 A worrying adverse effect of inhaling solvents from a plastic bag (8)

Down

1 Testing for this is necessary if there is a suggestion of the use of contaminated needles (3)

2 Increased dose needed to achieve same desired effect (9)

4 Drug taken to increase alertness and energy (12)

6 Pupil reaction when cocaine is taken (7)

61. Genetic Abnormalities I

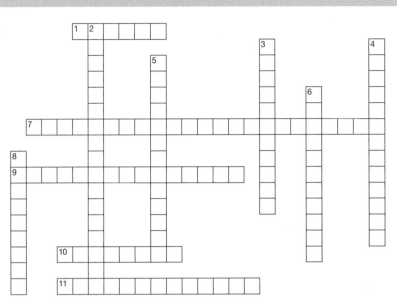

Across

1 Syndrome caused by trisomy of chromosome 13 (6)

7 Laboratory technique to amplify DNA samples (10,5,8)

9 Trisomy 18 with features of low birth weight, small jaw, overlapping fingers and cardiac defects (7,8)

10 Syndrome representing the second most common cause of severe learning difficulties (7,1)

11 Type of mutation inherited from the mother (13)

Down

2 Type of genetic abnormality responsible for neurofibromatosis and Huntington's disease (9,8)

3 Term for congenital anatomical malformation, usually with distinctive facial features (11)

4 Marrying someone who has descended from the same blood ancestor (13)

5 Trisomy 21 (5,8)

6 Physical feature of Turner's syndrome (4,7)

8 Gene that is not expressed in heterozygotes (9)

62. Genetic Abnormalities II

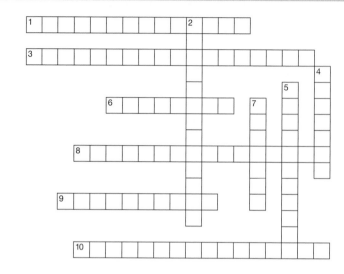

Across

1 Type of dwarfism caused by autosomal dominant genetic abnormality (14)

3 Assisting individuals and families cope with the diagnosis of a genetic disease (7,11)

6 Genetic disease mostly found in Eastern European Jews (3-5)

8 Serum levels measured as part of the triple test to screen for Down's syndrome (5,11)

9 Urethral defect associated with undescended testes (10)

10 Type of inheritance present in haemophilia A and B (1-6,9)

Down

2 Invasive technique used for karyotyping (13)

4 Syndrome with the presentation of elongated limbs and aneurysms (7)

5 Obese child with mental retardation in which the paternal chromosome is unexpressed or absent (6-5)

7 Chronic renal failure, sensorineural deafness and cataracts are all features of this inherited syndrome (7)

63. Complications of Down's Syndrome

Find 19 clinical features of Down's syndrome in the grid. Words can go horizontally, vertically and diagonally in all eight directions.

R	F	T	H	M	E	X	Y	L	Y	T	C	A	D	O	N	I	L	C	W	P	E	R
E	R	C	H	M	R	R	E	X	B	H	H	R	C	Y	T	N	K	R	L	P	B	P
S	K	E	P	X	U	S	S	N	T	Z	M	W	L	G	V	F	N	X	I	F	J	T
P	Z	F	L	L	S	I	A	R	M	K	G	K	T	L	W	N	K	C	M	C	Q	S
I	W	E	T	E	S	N	E	D	K	S	Q	F	R	Q	Z	C	A	M	W	R	T	B
R	N	D	D	A	I	G	S	H	T	T	I	K	L	T	K	N	M	D	B	O	M	N
A	C	L	C	R	F	L	I	J	Q	T	Y	D	K	A	T	L	T	R	P	T	C	M
T	H	A	B	N	L	E	D	T	G	Y	Y	M	I	H	T	G	R	S	M	A	M	R
O	P	T	M	I	A	P	S	D	T	M	W	M	I	O	H	O	D	L	I	X	H	L
R	N	P	R	N	R	A	R	K	E	T	Y	C	S	K	R	L	C	S	K	R	R	H
Y	J	E	K	G	B	L	E	B	V	A	F	V	P	S	E	Y	E	C	R	G	Y	B
I	C	S	N	D	E	M	M	M	L	O	F	C	L	I	E	R	H	M	I	P	G	K
N	D	R	V	I	P	A	I	D	L	P	G	N	F	K	T	N	X	T	O	P	C	V
F	L	A	Y	F	L	R	E	D	B	N	Q	H	E	A	D	H	T	T	O	R	U	G
E	L	L	B	F	A	C	H	T	C	J	S	K	L	S	L	N	O	R	L	P	H	T
C	X	U	W	I	P	R	Z	H	H	U	V	A	F	K	S	N	Q	Z	O	K	Y	B
T	Z	C	Y	C	W	E	L	X	R	P	N	B	J	H	I	G	G	T	P	H	K	H
I	L	I	M	U	O	A	A	B	Y	E	J	B	M	A	L	D	T	R	Y	Y	S	T
O	M	R	K	L	R	S	L	X	D	G	N	Z	D	H	N	B	F	J	K	J	N	W
N	D	T	Q	T	R	E	D	O	D	Y	N	K	S	T	C	A	R	A	T	A	C	R
S	F	N	T	I	A	Q	U	R	P	Y	T	N	D	R	D	L	Q	Y	Q	L	H	W
Z	H	E	J	E	N	D	T	T	M	Y	O	P	I	A	T	P	Q	T	N	J	Y	R
M	D	V	X	S	F	P	R	O	T	R	U	D	I	N	G	T	O	N	G	U	E	R

64. Causes of Developmental Delay

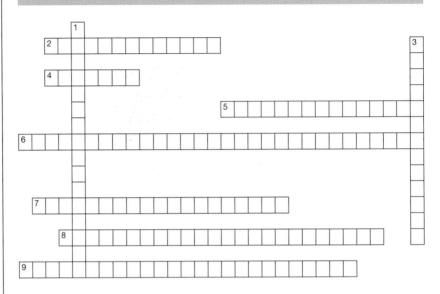

Across

2 Non-progressive intracranial lesion responsible for delayed motor development (8,5)

4 Child presenting with unkempt appearance, short stature and developmental delay (7)

5 Intrauterine infection (15)

6 Developmental delay as a result of deprivation of oxygen at birth (7,9,14)

7 Cause of an obese child with global developmental delay (6-5,8)

8 Uncommon cause of developmental delay since heel prick test introduced (10,14)

9 X-linked recessive condition with delayed walking and Gower's sign (8,8,9)

Down

1 Global developmental delay in a boy whose brother also has learning difficulties (7,1,8)

3 Global developmental delay in child with dysmorphic facial features, such as epicanthic fold of the eyelids (5,8)

65. Emotional and Behavioural Problems

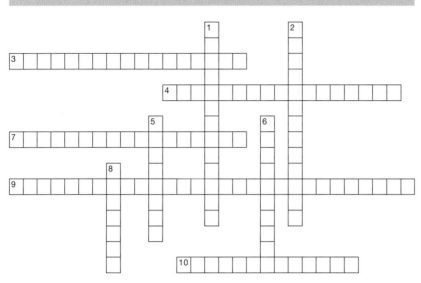

Across

3 Young children who become upset when a person they are attached to leaves (10,7)

4 Bed-wetting (9,8)

7 Mild form of autism (9,8)

9 Hyperkinetic syndrome (9,7,13)

10 Non-organic symptom with underlying emotional problems (13)

Down

1 Child exhales fully without taking another breath – this leads to cyanosis (6-7)

2 Lack of self-control in response to frustration, mainly seen in preschoolers (6,7)

5 Difficulty in learning to read (8)

6 Faecal soiling in inappropriate places in children over 4 years of age (10)

8 Technique to help overcome sleep disorders (7)

66. Causes of Short Stature

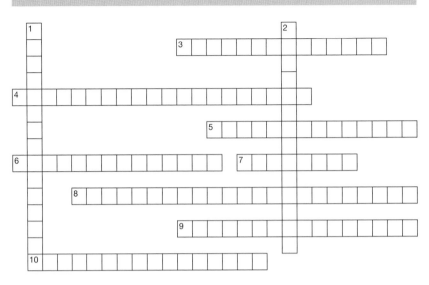

Across

3   Inherited disorder with features of shortened limbs and abnormally large skull (14)

4   Chronic disease where diagnosis becomes apparent looking at the urea and electrolyte levels (5,7,8)

5   Chronic disease that causes malabsorption resulting in poor growth as well as severe recurrent respiratory infections (6,8)

6   A child with pale, yellow-tinged skin complains of lethargy and intolerance to the cold (14)

7   Short stature but normal growth within parental height range (8)

8   Short, obese child with small genitalia and a history of difficult birth (6,7,10)

9   Investigations reveal glucocorticoid deficiency (8,8)

10 Non-organic cause of short stature (9,7)

Down

1   Poor growth in a girl with a webbed neck and widely spaced nipples (7,8)

2   Child with a history of diarrhoea and investigations reveal iron deficiency (7,7)

67. Disorders of Sexual Development

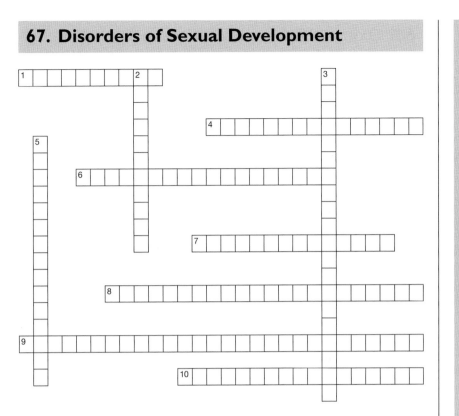

Across

1 Premature development of pubic hair (10)
4 Psychiatric diagnosis in which delayed puberty is a clinical sign (8,7)
6 Breast enlargement in female infants without other signs of puberty (9,9)
7 Difference between true precocious puberty and pseudo-precocious puberty in boys (10,4)
8 Inherited cause of true precocious puberty (6-8,8)
9 Autosomal recessive disorder causing pseudo-precocious puberty (10,7,11)
10 Inherited disease with benign growths on skin associated with the early onset of puberty (17)

Down

2 Most likely location for space-occupying CNS tumour that causes precocious puberty (11)
3 47XXY chromosome in men with undeveloped testicles (12,8)
5 Delayed puberty in which the karyotype is 45XO (7,8)

68. Organic Causes of Failure to Thrive

Find 21 causes of failure to thrive in the grid. Words can go horizontally, vertically and diagonally in all eight directions.

K	L	G	V	B	D	K	E	C	N	A	R	E	L	O	T	N	I	E	S	O	T	C	A	L	K	K	T
A	I	S	A	L	P	R	E	P	Y	H	L	A	N	E	R	D	A	L	A	T	I	N	E	G	N	O	C
A	I	M	E	A	N	A	Y	C	N	E	I	C	I	F	E	D	N	O	R	I	J	F	H	X	C	R	Z
W	C	R	D	J	R	L	G	M	J	R	S	U	T	I	L	L	E	M	S	E	T	E	B	A	I	D	L
Q	W	F	R	E	N	A	L	T	U	B	U	L	A	R	A	C	I	D	O	S	I	S	N	R	D	R	Q
C	J	X	Q	G	Z	C	N	O	I	T	C	E	F	N	I	T	C	A	R	T	Y	R	A	N	I	R	U
Z	P	D	L	R	Y	N	B	T	X	M	K	G	Z	R	Z	N	D	L	G	Z	L	C	J	P	C	J	F
K	K	E	M	O	R	D	N	Y	S	S	R	E	N	R	U	T	L	R	C	B	L	V	V	D	M	B	L
D	E	S	A	E	S	I	D	T	R	A	E	H	L	A	T	I	N	E	G	N	O	C	L	P	K	T	V
C	S	U	S	O	T	A	M	E	H	T	Y	R	E	S	U	P	U	L	C	I	M	E	T	S	Y	S	Q
Q	Y	T	L	Y	K	Q	J	R	V	Z	H	P	Z	L	Q	M	M	C	D	N	N	M	R	T	C	K	G
Q	F	S	M	G	A	S	T	R	O	O	E	S	O	P	H	A	G	E	A	L	R	E	F	L	U	X	T
Y	L	Y	T	Q	N	C	T	N	V	G	W	Z	Q	R	R	K	M	H	L	R	M	T	T	K	L	N	H
T	W	K	U	I	B	Z	D	R	M	D	G	M	X	B	C	E	Y	Q	I	N	Z	K	H	M	L	Y	M
R	K	R	B	T	C	M	G	L	T	N	H	W	F	O	B	L	C	Z	V	V	R	V	R	R	S	N	S
G	D	N	E	Z	T	F	B	P	B	R	Y	F	E	K	D	L	Z	N	Q	P	E	C	E	L	W	H	I
Z	T	K	R	K	G	W	I	F	T	R	H	L	D	X	L	P	N	J	A	H	N	S	A	J	Q	C	D
T	R	P	C	R	X	D	Y	B	T	J	I	Z	G	D	Y	L	V	D	E	C	A	P	T	H	M	L	I
N	N	I	U	C	T	Y	N	L	R	A	N	T	F	B	P	H	N	A	N	E	L	C	R	T	Q	P	O
D	T	L	L	B	M	K	M	C	C	O	L	B	Z	H	R	R	R	T	S	A	F	R	D	Y	G	D	R
K	L	T	O	M	V	N	T	D	C	H	S	Y	Q	K	T	T	Q	I	R	G	A	G	F	M	R	D	Y
N	Y	F	S	B	P	Y	I	P	J	Y	R	I	R	R	F	M	D	B	T	L	I	J	Q	B	N	X	H
N	L	E	I	R	L	S	J	C	M	C	X	M	S	A	J	S	E	C	J	N	L	K	H	J	D	W	T
G	N	L	S	F	E	N	K	Q	R	N	R	T	I	Q	N	R	Y	H	C	Z	U	W	X	W	W	M	O
K	Q	C	T	A	N	F	R	L	K	T	P	L	V	H	E	R	T	T	C	R	R	Y	T	L	T	F	P
J	H	Q	S	M	L	L	T	W	Q	Q	U	Q	O	C	R	M	Y	K	C	J	E	L	H	P	Q	G	Y
X	C	E	Z	K	M	F	M	L	Q	R	Y	R	T	H	X	B	F	T	N	W	J	M	R	Q	F	D	H
F	L	T	W	K	H	Z	B	C	E	Q	C	Y	G	W	T	J	G	K	R	R	M	C	N	D	V	V	L

69. Neonatal Examination

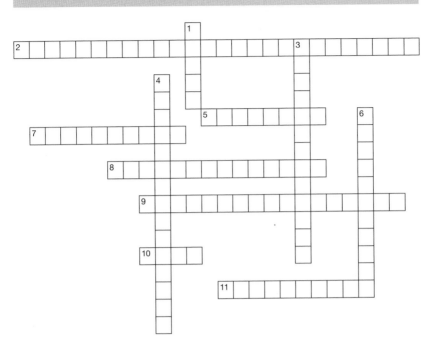

Across

2 Red patches in the eye associated with pressure changes in childbirth (15,11)

5 Manoeuvre to detect dislocation of the hip (8)

7 Birth defect of the urethra (10)

8 Cause of a negative red reflex of the retina (14)

9 Cause of blue skin patches in dark-skinned neonates (9,4,4)

10 Reflex when the baby's head is tilted backwards (4)

11 Soft part of the head palpated (10)

Down

1 Pearly white spots on the nose and cheeks (5)

3 Sign of cystic fibrosis in a newborn baby (8,5)

4 Circumference measuring the head size (15)

6 Birth defect found on examination of the mouth (5,6)

70. Developmental Examination

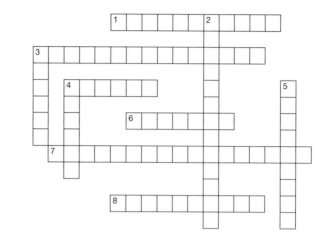

Across

1 Test used to assess a baby's hearing (11)
3 Term used when a child's growth is less than normal (7,2,6)
4 Grasp reflex using the whole hand (6)
6 Clinical sign when pulled to sitting before head control is established (4,3)
7 Examination technique in which the baby is held in the prone position (7,10)
8 Misalignment of the eyes (10)

Down

2 Cause of asymmetrical response to Moro reflex (8,5)
3 Poor limb tone (6)
4 Grasp reflex using finger and thumb tested in babies 10 months old (6)
5 Age a baby should be able to sit-up (3,6)

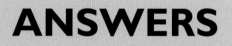

ANSWERS

1. Nutrition

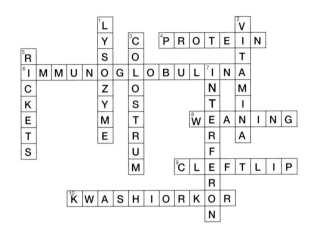

Anti-infective properties of breast milk	Comments
Immunoglobulin A	Main maternal antibody, particularly through colostrum (yellow fluid secreted in first few days of birth)
Lysozyme	Enzyme that breaks down bacterial cell walls
Interferon	Has antiviral properties
Lactoferrin	Iron binds to bacteria inhibiting replication

There is much higher content of protein in cow's milk than in human milk.

If a baby is born with a cleft lip, breast-feeding should be avoided.

The term 'weaning' describes a baby who has been started on solid foods as opposed to being solely fed on breast milk.

Rickets is a bone disorder occurring as a result of vitamin D or calcium deficiency. The lack of vitamin A manifests as visual impairment and stunted growth. Kwashiorkor is a form of protein malnutrition with typical features of a distended abdomen, muscle wasting and flaking skin.

2. Causes of Vomiting

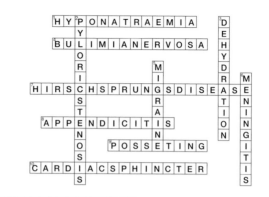

Disorder	Comments
Pyloric stenosis	In babies 4–8 weeks old; projectile, non-bilious vomiting, associated with subsequent hunger
Gastroenteritis	In all age-groups; presents with vomiting and diarrhoea, sometimes leads to dehydration; mostly viral in the UK; bacterial causes more severe vomiting and diarrhoea
Gastro-oesophageal reflux	Common in <1-year-olds; occurs when cardiac sphincter is incompetent or where there is largely liquid intake
Intestinal obstruction	Examples include intussusception, volvulus, and Hirschsprung's disease; presents with vomiting (sometimes bile-stained), abdominal pain, distension and constipation
Appendicitis	In >2-year-olds; initially presents with central abdominal pain and vomiting
Meningitis	Presents with vomiting in conjunction with fever, neck stiffness, photophobia and bulging fontanelles in babies
Migraine	In older children; symptoms of chronic unilateral headaches, which may be preceded by visual aura and associated with vomiting
Increased intracranial pressure	Such as caused by CNS tumour – vomiting and headache early in the morning
Bulimia nervosa	Mostly older children; binge-eating followed by self-induced vomiting
Metabolic disorders	Hyponatraemia; ketoacidosis; hyperammoniaemia

'Posseting' is the term referring to the regurgitation of milk after a baby has been fed.

3. Acute Abdominal Pain

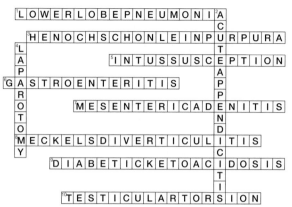

The crossword answers, reading as placed in the grid:

- LOWERLOBEPNEUMONIA
- HENOCHSCHONLEINPURPURA
- INTUSSUSCEPTION
- GASTROENTERITIS
- MESENTERICADENITIS
- MECKELSDIVERTICULITIS
- DIABETICKETOACIDOSIS
- TESTICULARTORSION
- Down: LAPAROTOMY, ACUTEAPPENDICITIS

Cause	Comments
Acute appendicitis	Central abdominal pain radiating to right iliac fossa, anorexia, vomiting, low-grade fever, tenderness at McBurney's point in the right iliac fossa
Mesenteric adenitis	Features of URTI – fever, pharyngitis, nausea, right iliac fossa pain that shifts with position changes
Gastroenteritis	Diarrhoea, vomiting, abdominal pain, dehydration. In severe cases – dysentery
Meckel's diverticulitis	In <10-year-olds; central abdominal pain with rectal bleeding
Intussusception	Mostly in infants of 3–12 months old; typically episodes of severe, colicky abdominal pain and vomiting, 'redcurrant jelly' stools, sausage-shaped mass in right upper quadrant
Henoch–Schönlein purpura	Symmetrical purpuric rash on buttocks and lower extremities, arthritis (knees, ankles), colicky abdominal pain and melaena; microscopic haematuria and proteinuria
Testicular torsion	Referred abdominal pain and firm, tender, scrotal swelling; can lead to strangulation, necrosis and atrophy of the testes
Diabetic ketoacidosis	Abdominal pain, Kussmaul breathing (slow, deep breathing), ketotic breath
Lower lobe pneumonia	Referred abdominal pain along with symptoms of chest pain, purulent sputum, dyspnoea and fever

Laparotomy is a surgical incision into the abdominal cavity for diagnostic and therapeutic purposes, indicated if the cause of abdominal pain is unknown, principally if there are signs of peritonitis.

4. Causes of Recurrent Abdominal Pain

Word List: abdominal migraine; calculus; cholecystitis; constipation; Crohn's disease; gastritis; giardiasis; hepatitis; intussusception; irritable bowel syndrome; malrotation; non-ulcer dyspepsia; ovarian tumour; pancreatitis; pelvic inflammatory disease; peptic ulcer; porphyria; urinary tract infection.

C	M	A	L	R	O	T	A	T	I	O	N	T	P	X	R	Z	H	T	L	L	M	P	L	E
B	A	T	G	R	T	Q	T	Q	R	L	R	E	B	L	K	L	F	G	B	X	L	G	V	S
N	L	L	V	C	M	M	M	L	K	T	P	C	O	N	S	T	I	P	A	T	I	O	N	A
Y	O	D	C	N	V	Y	C	T	D	Y	G	N	R	M	E	Y	T	F	W	G	Q	C	T	E
D	R	I	B	U	P	R	W	V	I	L	N	M	L	R	M	C	M	Q	R	I	Y	L	Q	S
M	W	R	T	F	L	R	X	C	L	R	J	H	B	B	O	C	R	D	U	A	G	N	X	I
Q	L	N	L	P	T	U	U	N	R	H	B	K	G	D	F	Y	F	S	O	R	G	O	Z	D
D	L	P	D	W	E	L	S	H	L	M	T	S	Q	C	D	E	T	I	M	D	L	N	Y	Y
S	J	C	Y	B	C	O	H	R	G	G	I	B	R	J	J	X	H	T	U	I	N	U	R	R
D	I	P	R	E	P	P	S	L	N	I	N	Q	Y	Y	M	X	I	T	A	R	L	T	C
Z	K	T	R	O	F	N	T	U	I	T	Q	P	A	M	S	L	G	T	N	S	L	C	P	T
L	G	L	I	H	H	Q	X	R	S	G	N	P	M	K	L	N	R	A	A	I	C	E	P	A
X	K	B	N	T	X	N	T	B	M	S	C	L	T	H	E	K	V	E	I	S	R	R	W	M
W	L	N	K	L	A	S	S	L	D	I	U	V	F	T	W	P	K	F	R	L	L	D	C	M
P	Q	L	N	Y	A	R	T	D	M	V	B	T	B	R	C	N	V	C	A	X	L	Y	N	A
P	N	P	K	G	L	K	E	I	T	D	J	N	R	B	L	T	N	V	Q	W	S	Z	L
D	L	M	P	M	T	B	A	H	Q	S	N	V	P	I	E	X	X	A	O	G	K	P	C	F
P	L	R	L	G	H	N	R	W	J	C	E	H	H	H	L	V	Q	P	T	V	G	E	Y	N
L	L	R	N	D	I	Y	V	R	K	M	Y	A	N	X	B	F	J	R	J	P	D	F	T	I
M	J	T	F	M	C	R	F	M	R	R	Z	V	S	M	A	P	J	X	K	L	W	S	X	C
Z	M	V	O	K	H	M	Q	O	I	F	T	K	V	E	T	V	V	B	F	H	B	I	C	I
B	W	D	W	R	L	P	J	A	Q	T	R	L	B	X	I	K	H	Y	N	Y	P	A	T	V
N	B	T	N	O	I	T	C	E	F	N	I	T	C	A	R	T	Y	R	A	N	I	R	U	L
A	K	J	Y	C	N	R	D	H	L	D	N	Z	W	R	R	T	K	X	Z	Y	N	C	Y	E
V	S	I	T	I	T	S	Y	C	E	L	O	H	C	F	I	T	N	X	P	M	G	C	J	F

The term 'recurrent abdominal pain' is used when the pain occurs on 3 or more occasions within 3 months. A small minority of recurrent abdominal complaints from children are organic.

System	Disorders
Gastrointestinal	Crohn's disease; constipation; gastritis; giardiasis; irritable bowel syndrome; malrotation; intussusception; non-ulcer dyspepsia; peptic ulcer
Hepatobiliary	Hepatitis; cholecystitis
Pancreatic	Pancreatitis
Genitourinary	Urinary tract infection; calculus
Gynaecological	Ovarian tumour; pelvic inflammatory disease
Other	Abdominal migraine; porphyria

5. Causes of Constipation

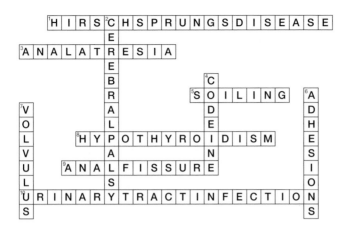

Disorder	Comments
Anal atresia	In neonates; absent or abnormally placed anus, often associated with fistulae
Hirschsprung's disease	In neonates; aganglionic segment of bowel; features include delayed passage of meconium and distended abdomen; later, constipation with bile-stained vomit
Volvulus	Abnormal twisting of bowel resulting in obstruction; symptoms of acute obstruction – abdominal pain, vomiting and constipation
Adhesions	Post-surgery complication; symptoms of acute obstruction
Neurological disorders	Mytonic dystrophy, cerebral palsy
Drugs	Codeine, antidepressants
Others	Hypothyroidism, hypercalcaemia

Urinary tract infection may occur when constipation is severe enough to obstruct the urinary stream, allowing urine to accumulate in the bladder for longer periods.

Soiling refers to constipation with overflow or the involuntary and inappropriate passage of stools.

The passage of hard stools predisposes an individual to anal fissures.

6. Causes of Chronic Diarrhoea

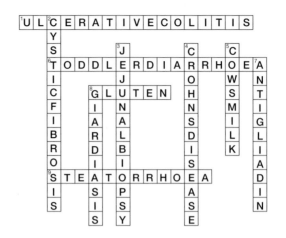

Disorder	Comments
Toddler diarrhoea	In preschoolers; 3–4 times a day of diarrhoea consisting of undigested food particles in a thriving child
Coeliac disease	Gluten-sensitive malabsorption disorder; symptoms of steatorrhoea (pale fatty stools), failure to thrive and muscle wasting; screening test using antiendomysial and IgA antigliadin antibodies; diagnosis based on positive jejunal biopsy results
Food allergies	For example cow's milk, nuts; often family history of atopic diseases; symptoms of diarrhoea, failure to thrive and sometimes vomiting
Crohn's disease	In older children and adolescents; symptoms of growth failure with pubertal delay associated with bouts of abdominal pain and diarrhoea, perianal ulcers and fissures
Ulcerative colitis	Rarer than Crohn's disease; symptoms of bloody diarrhoea, colicky abdominal pain, weight loss, and some cases of skin lesions and arthritis
Giardiasis	Protozoan infection acquired mostly through foreign travel; symptoms include chronic steatorrhoea, weight loss and abdominal pain; cysts seen on microscopy

7. Gastroenteritis

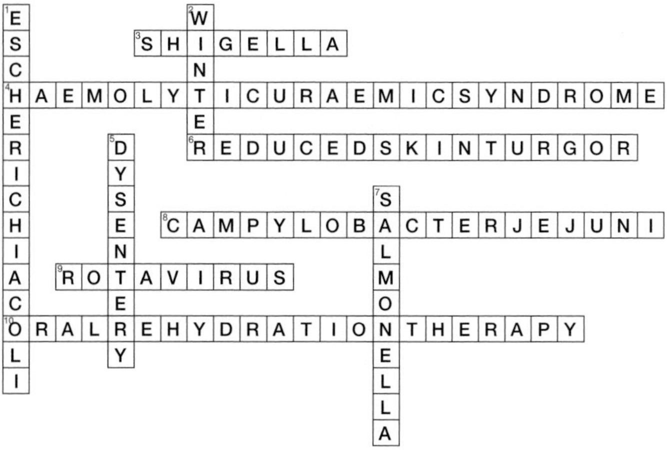

Pathogen	*Comments*
Rotavirus	Commonest cause in developed world in infants; occurs mostly in winter; symptoms of severe watery diarrhoea, vomiting and high fever
Campylobacter jejuni	After consumption of infected chicken or milk; symptoms of severe abdominal pain and bloody diarrhoea
Salmonella	Common sources – undercooked eggs and poultry; symptoms of loose diarrhoea, vomiting and systemic upset
Shigella	Affects preschoolers; symptoms of dysentery, high fever, some pain and occasionally febrile convulsions
Escherichia coli	Affects <2-year-olds; common sources – contaminated meat and raw cow's milk; symptoms of profuse watery diarrhoea, vomiting; can lead to haemolytic uraemic syndrome – microangiopathic haemolytic anaemia, thrombocytopenia, acute renal failure

Dysentery can be defined as blood and mucus in the stools indicating inflammation of the lower part of the intestinal tract.

Signs of dehydration include sunken eyes, reduced skin turgor, dry mucous membranes and poor capillary refill. Mild dehydration (<5% weight loss) is managed with oral rehydration therapy, whereas in cases of 5–10% weight loss, intravenous fluids are recommended in the hospital.

8. Causes of Rectal Bleeding

Word List: anal fissure; *Campylobacter jejuni*; Crohn's disease; *Entamoeba histolytica*; haemolytic uraemic syndrome; haemorrhoids; Henoch–Schönlein purpura; intussusception; Meckel's diverticulum; milk allergy; prolapse; rectal polyp; *Salmonella*; sexual abuse; *Shigella*; trauma; ulcerative colitis.

Cause	Disorders
Infective	*Campylobacter jejuni*; *Entamoeba histolytica*; *Salmonella*; *Shigella*
Non-infective	Anal fissure; Crohn's disease; haemolytic uraemic syndrome; haemorrhoids; Henoch–Schönlein purpura; intussusception; Meckel's diverticulum; milk allergy; prolapse; rectal polyp; sexual abuse; trauma; ulcerative colitis

Typical presentation of bacterial gastrointestinal infections is blood and mucus in the stools. Intussusception should be suspected when rectal bleeding is noticed in neonates.

9. Genital Disorders

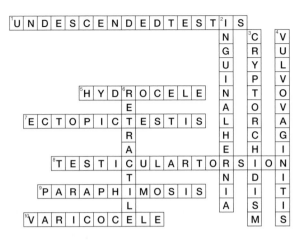

Crossword solution:

- 1. UNDESCENDED TESTIS
- 5. HYDROCELE
- 7. ECTOPIC TESTIS
- 8. TESTICULAR TORSION
- 9. PARAPHIMOSIS
- 10. VARICOCELE

Down:
- 2. INGUINAL HERNIA
- 3. CRYPTORCHIDISM
- 4. VULVOVAGINITIS

Disorder	Comments
Cryptorchidism	Undescended testis – more prevalent in premature babies; testis impalpable in scrotum but can be gently manipulated from inguinal canal to scrotum Ectopic testis – testis outside normal descent; on examination, testis cannot be manipulated into scrotum
Retractile	Testis can be gently manipulated into scrotum from inguinal canal but returns to original position because of hyperactivity of cremaster muscle
Inguinal hernia	Reducible scrotal swelling that is more prominent on coughing and straining; if strangulated – severe acute pain in scrotum
Paraphimosis	Irretractible foreskin behind glans penis; usually can be reduced under anaesthetic
Hydrocele	Painless fluid-filled swelling in scrotum that transilluminates in the dark; usually resolved by 12 months of age
Varicocele	Tortuous veins around testes; mainly in adolescents; usually asymptomatic but can cause dragging or aching sensation in scrotum
Testicular torsion	More common in infants <1 year of age and in adolescence; acute, severe pain in scrotum, groin and lower abdomen, and swelling in testicle associated with nausea and dizziness

The presentation of vulvovaginitis is pain in the vulva and vaginal discharge.

10. Renal Diseases

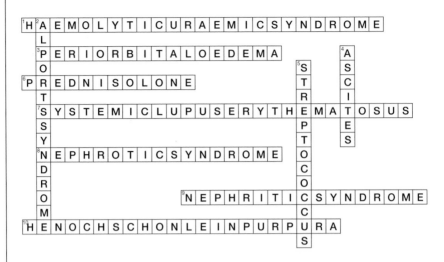

Disorder	Comments
Nephrotic syndrome	Clinical features include generalized oedema (in particular facial, periorbital and scrotal), ascites and pleural effusion; investigations reveal hypoalbuminaemia, hypercholesterolaemia and excessive proteinuria; prednisolone is first-line treatment
Nephritic syndrome	Glomerulonephritis; main causes include streptococci, Henoch–Schönlein purpura, haemolytic uraemic syndrome, and occasionally SLE; clinical features of periorbital oedema, hypertension and loin pain; investigations reveal haematuria, proteinuria and elevated serum creatinine
Henoch–Schönlein purpura	Clinical features of purpuric symmetrical rash over extensor surfaces and buttocks, arthralgia and abdominal pain; investigations show haematuria and proteinuria (from glomerulitis)
Haemolytic uraemic syndrome	Mostly following bloody diarrhoea caused by *E. coli* infection; main features include acute renal failure, haemolytic anaemia and thrombocytopenia
Alport's syndrome	Inherited disorder; chronic kidney failure with ocular and hearing problems

11. Urinary Tract Infections

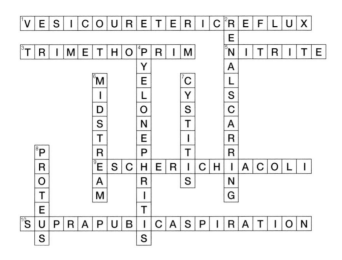

Escherichia coli, a part of the bowel flora, is the most common causative agent to infect the urinary tract. Another common causative organism is *Proteus*, affecting boys more than girls.

The congenital anomaly, vesicoureteric reflux, is a predisposing factor to acquiring a UTI because the reflux, from the bladder to the ureter, causes urine to stagnate, making it an optimal environment for bacteria to reproduce.

Neonates tend to present with non-specific symptoms, such as vomiting and fever, whereas older children have features of more classical UTIs, which include frequency, enuresis, dysuria and fever (cystitis). If the infection has spread to the kidneys, known as pyelonephritis, the child may experience loin pain.

Age group	Method of collection
<1-year-olds	Bag sample, suprapubic aspiration (in urgent cases)
Preschoolers	Clean catch sample
Older children	Midstream sample

Urine dipstick tests can be done at the bedside to detect for the presence of nitrites and leucocytes indicating infection.

Management includes trimethoprim along with fluid intake, unless there are further complications, in which case a broad-spectrum antibiotic may be more suitable. Ineffective treatment can result in renal scarring, but this is rare.

12. Causes of Haematuria

Word List: Alport's syndrome; anticoagulants; cyclophosphamide; exercise; glomerulonephritis; haemolytic uraemic syndrome; Henoch–Schönlein purpura; hypercalciuria; IgA nephropathy; polycystic kidney disease; renal vascular thrombosis; sickle-cell anaemia; stones; systemic lupus erythematosus; thrombocytopenia; trauma; urinary tract infection; Wilms' tumour.

H	H	N	N	S	H	D	B	R	A	L	P	O	R	T	S	S	Y	N	D	R	O	M	E	Q	P
A	M	J	W	Y	W	F	P	X	T	M	L	L	L	X	Q	B	H	K	V	W	W	R	Y	M	K
E	K	W	Q	S	N	N	J	G	R	Z	D	K	N	K	B	X	G	N	J	P	H	K	G	E	W
M	P	A	T	I	S	T	T	M	T	T	K	C	Y	R	D	K	N	F	M	T	X	M	D	T	J
O	O	R	T	E	I	N	R	G	L	O	M	E	R	U	L	O	N	E	P	H	R	I	T	I	S
L	L	U	G	M	S	O	L	Y	R	T	W	R	T	H	H	R	Z	F	Z	B	M	K	M	T	D
Y	Y	F	C	I	O	I	P	D	K	W	N	M	N	J	W	B	C	F	L	A	V	M	G	K	Z
T	O	F	D	O	E	T	L	E	Q	T	M	Z	B	P	P	J	H	H	H	B	K	H	N	T	K
I	Y	L	K	L	M	O	R	X	M	N	M	N	K	Z	R	F	N	P	P	A	K	Q	T	A	K
O	S	F	L	U	O	E	H	E	R	W	C	Y	X	N	L	M	S	Z	N	H	R	T	I	J	Z
U	T	N	C	F	R	R	Z	R	W	J	H	B	H	A	V	O	R	T	X	T	T	N	M	P	K
F	I	I	K	U	H	N	K	O	T	T	G	X	M	H	B	I	K	N	D	E	W	Q	H	T
A	O	E	J	S	I	I	Z	I	B	F	R	U	X	P	A	C	N	L	R	P	G	L	Y	W	B
E	K	L	K	E	R	I	T	S	T	D	A	O	O	O	R	C	X	O	M	K	W	W	W	P
M	I	N	L	R	A	O	X	E	X	R	L	S	A	R	M	O	T	M	V	B	V	L	Z	N
I	D	O	G	Y	L	A	L	M	T	N	C	G	W	Y	R	T	L	D	B	V	Y	J
O	N	H	R	T	U	F	M	D	M	Y	K	U	N	I	O	A	X	H	F	L	J	T	D	R
S	E	O	N	H	O	T	T	L	C	L	L	L	M	O	N	M	N	R	L	N	J	Z	Q
Y	Y	S	B	E	S	Y	C	Y	R	A	D	M	B	Y	J	E	O	C	H	E	H	P	T	R
N	D	H	F	M	A	R	J	R	N	O	S	M	Q	N	R	R	S	T	W	N	Q	P	T
D	I	O	F	A	V	A	X	T	G	T	O	M	L	L	C	K	K	Z	Q	U	M	A	M	R
F	S	O	T	T	L	N	S	K	U	R	C	B	W	M	W	M	L	N	N	M	R	T	G	M
O	E	N	T	O	A	I	Y	M	N	H	G	F	K	T	C	L	G	M	K	G	C	K	J	I
M	A	E	C	S	N	R	O	W	T	D	J	Q	L	R	G	W	K	T	M	N	C	B	L	A	Q
E	S	H	G	U	E	U	A	I	M	E	A	N	A	L	L	E	C	E	L	K	C	I	S	Z	T
W	E	T	L	S	R	M	L	R	R	Y	W	V	F	L	F	Q	Z	M	K	V	G	M	M	D	D

When blood is visible in the urine, the disorder is known as macroscopic haematuria. Microscopic haematuria can be detected on dipsticks or microscopy but cannot be seen by the naked eye.

System	Disorders
Renal	Glomerulonephritis; IgA nephropathy; Alport's syndrome; Henoch–Schönlein purpura; haemolytic uraemic syndrome; polycystic kidney disease; Wilms' tumour; SLE; renal vascular thrombosis
Urinary tract	Urinary tract infection; stones; hypercalciuria; cyclophosphamide
Haematological	Thrombocytopenia; sickle-cell anaemia; anticoagulants
Others	Exercise; trauma

13. Causes of Acute Renal Failure

Word List: acute tubular necrosis; burns; dehydration; gastroenteritis; glomerulonephritis; haemolytic uraemic syndrome; haemorrhage; heart failure; interstitial nephritis; nephrotic syndrome; papillary necrosis; pyelonephritis; renal calculi; renal vein thrombosis; respiratory distress syndrome; sepsis.

```
E M O R D N Y S S S E R T S I D Y R O T A R I P S E R
M D Q R D R Y T X X F F N V G L Z T B G D T X F Z N Q
Q E M O R D N Y S C I M E A R U C I T Y L O M E A H R
V N S K N F V K Y D C Y W W F T K Q Y W M Z D H M L V
X K L K P D K L R J F C N F D H X M H X V H F M P Z
P L K Z S P V L K N L M K R C K N W M B C L Q N P K G
V N F T Q Q T W K N Q D E H Y D R A T I O N S P V Z L
M J N M D C R K Q Z M F P N K V K N W H R T T F R O
Y D Y M F S H C R N T G F Q M L C H T C K P K E Q M
R X R F E W E M E L K W A J Z M X X B Z A P N F W E
T E E F C R R P N M W Z S Q M R Q F V A P N W R
T M N G X G U V S V R D G W W F H C N L G E D D U
M O A H L T L L K K A G H K R Z L V G X T M L
L R L M K M K G T S L K D E O V E N A J Y Y R O
Y D C Z X M J M X A T P G U N L A E Z H Z V C F N N
L N A J B Y W V B R V N O B R W N N R M R L N K S E
F Y L C N W T T N C C B U Y R T L M J M N P
Y S C G M K C P H L Z E R N K H T O Z V E Z Z C R R H
N C U Y Q B L T R T Y Q E A R M M E M X N R F R K U R
Z L K Y T N Z V P V C P O E E T Z T T B Z P B
Q I L H D N K Y G R N M R A H B T M U T Y F T R F T
M O M V H V K K N O G B D H Z K T L W R C Y D H R I
W R G G L M T N S T O X H K W V R W Q B L A F V K S S
Y H R X F L W K S X Y Y T K Z H V D Y G T Q F N Q N
G P P T K X S R L J R W M Q R R L L F C D L T W C G
B E H Z N L L S R W M L L R L Z M H T B N J R L M K M
R N H I N T E R S T I T I A L N E P H R I T I S N R F
```

When the kidneys suddenly lose the ability to function, it is known as acute renal failure. Consequently, the kidneys can no longer remove waste products or maintain the fluid and electrolyte balance of the body. The main cause of acute renal failure in the developed world is haemolytic uraemic syndrome.

Classification	Causes
Prerenal	Burns; dehydration; gastroenteritis; haemorrhage; heart failure; sepsis; respiratory distress syndrome
Renal	Haemolytic uraemic syndrome; acute tubular necrosis; glomerulonephritis; interstitial nephritis; nephrotic syndrome; papillary necrosis; pyelonephritis; renal vein thrombosis
Postrenal	Renal calculi

14. Headaches

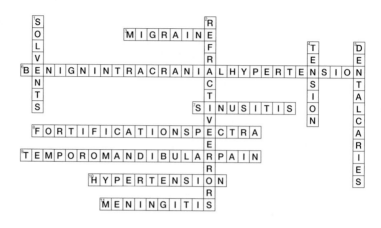

Disorder	Comments
Migraine	Unilateral throbbing headaches sometimes accompanied by visual aura – bright flashing lights, fortification spectra (zig-zag hallucination), nausea/vomiting and photophobia; triggered by anxiety, lack of sleep and certain foods
Tension headache	Band-like headache with fatigue and dizziness that comes on gradually throughout the day
Meningitis	Headache with photophobia and irritability, neck stiffness often absent in infants
Benign intracranial hypertension	In overweight female adolescents; throbbing headache worse in morning accompanied by gradual loss of vision and nausea; on examination – papilloedema
Sinusitis	Headache on waking up in morning, facial pain and rhinorrhoea
Temporomandibular pain	Referred pain, from orofacial area, on chewing and speaking
Refractive errors	Poor eyesight associated with headache; can be corrected by prescription glasses
Solvents	Sniffed or breathed-in, mainly by adolescent boys; consequent effects of drowsiness and headaches
Dental caries	Referred pain from tooth decay; tooth sensitivity on eating hot or cold food
Hypertension	Encephalopathy – serious and rare cause of headaches

15. Causes of Funny Turns

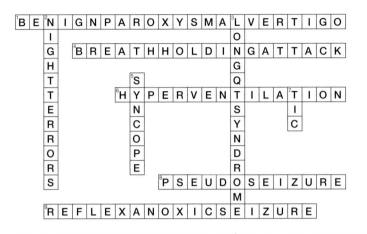

```
B E N I G N P A R O X Y S M A L V E R T I G O
  I                           O
  G   B R E A T H H O L D I N G A T T A C K
  H                           G
  T         S                 Q
  T         H Y P E R V E N T I L A T I O N
  E         N                 S         I
  R         C                 Y         C
  R         O                 N
  O         P                 D
  R         E                 R
  S             P S E U D O S E I Z U R E
                              M
  R E F L E X A N O X I C S E I Z U R E
```

Causes	Comments
Breath-holding	In preschoolers; angry child holds breath in expiration, leads to cyanosis and sometimes loss of consciousness
Reflex anoxic seizures	In preschoolers; episodes of pallor and loss of consciousness – may lead to a limp, then stiffness of the limbs, jerking of arms and legs brought on by fear and minor trauma
Benign paroxysmal vertigo	Episodes of imbalance, nausea and nystagmus with normal consciousness
Night terrors	In preschoolers; whilst asleep – dilated pupils, confused, unresponsive, unlikely to remember episode
Syncope	Mainly adolescents; vasovagal faint in particular after standing for long periods
Pseudoseizure	Mimics epileptic seizure, normal EEG
Hyperventilation	Triggered by anxiety; symptoms of over-breathing, results in lightheadedness and tingling in hands, feet and lips
Long-QT syndrome (rare)	Cardiac arrhythmia; fainting after exercise or anger

A tic is an abrupt involuntary movement that usually involves the muscles of the face and shoulders.

16. Causes of Hearing Impairment

Word List: aminoglycosides; birth asphyxia; cleft palate; cytomegalovirus; Down's syndrome; encephalitis; foreign body; hyperbilirubinaemia; kernicterus; meningitis; otosclerosis; prematurity; rubella; secretory otitis media; Treacher Collins syndrome; wax.

R	N	H	T	Z	H	Y	N	M	T	Y	M	R	L	R	G	P	K	X	T	X	F	E
Z	J	F	S	U	R	I	V	O	L	A	G	E	M	O	T	Y	C	R	P	D	Q	M
Q	P	O	F	G	M	A	Z	L	F	K	N	R	C	N	P	L	L	F	K	C	L	O
Q	V	R	Y	M	D	I	R	Y	W	R	K	K	R	H	F	N	X	B	Q	N	D	R
P	B	E	T	Z	H	D	G	J	T	F	N	Q	Q	M	R	F	X	Y	D	N	E	D
R	D			M	S	E	D	I	S	O	C	Y	L	G	O	N	I	M	A	N	M	N
L	B	G	R	T	M	M	F	B	F	D	K	T	Y	M	R	Q	H	G	C	Z	T	Y
V	W	N	U	N	M	S	W	C	Q	L	Z	L	R	U	A	T	J	E	D	W	P	S
R	V	B	T	L	B	I	G	Q	L	W	L	W	B	Y	Z	L	P	D	A	F	L	S
Z	C	O	A	Q	V	T	L	R	M	T	N	H	Y	F	H	L	M	S	X	N
T	H	D	M	X	L	I	L	L	Y	B	L	S	T	R	A	K	X	E	U	T	Y
C	H	Y	E	F	K	T	J	R	H	L	D	G	S	L	W	D	R	B	L	F	L
P	C	T	R	C	Z	O	R	D	A	L	C	N	L	K	H	Q	E	Z	L	U	X	L
H	W	N	P	L	X	Y	R	V	T	P	D	T	F	P	N	T	D	C	H	F	R	O
C	M	W	J	E	G	R	V	L	N	W	T	S	R	C	L	T	N	T	M	C
T	Z	M	L	F	Z	O	Y	Q	N	S	A	N	X	X	R	W	R	Y	W	R
N	B	W	M	T	N	T	J	D	P	B	H	N	J	T	J	M	Q	X	W	T	E
K	V	D	T	P	C	E	D	N	Y	T	T	R	X	W	V	D	P	K	M	T	K	H
C	N	M	K	A	T	R	H	K	R	R	E	P	H	T	L	H	D	W	C	E	J	C
K	X	K	N	L	T	C	M	N	K	D	Q	J	L	T	W	T	B	J	C	P	A
W	N	L	R	A	N	E	B	N	N	K	D	Q	T	T	Q	N	T	K	T	R	B	E
K	Z	K	Q	T	L	S	M	E	N	I	N	G	I	T	I	S	V	J	F	G	T	R
R	X	V	N	E	V	D	C	T	O	S	C	L	E	R	O	S	I	S	T	P	T	T

It is more common to find hearing impairment due to conductive hearing loss rather than sensorineural problems. Generally, the main cause of deafness in children is secretory otitis media (glue ear).

Type	Causes
Conductive	Secretory otitis media; Down's syndrome; cleft palate; Treacher Collins syndrome; foreign body; wax
Sensorineural	Prematurity; cytomegalovirus; rubella; prematurity; birth asphyxia; kernicterus; encephalitis; meningitis; ototoxic drugs, e.g. aminoglycosides

17. Bacterial Meningitis

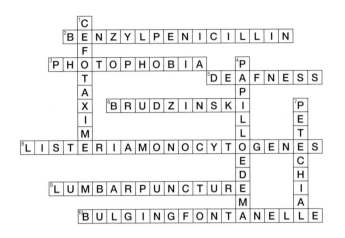

Bacteria that cause meningitis in children include *Neisseria meningitides*, *Haemophilus influenzae* and *Listeria monocytogenes* (in neonates).

Symptoms	Signs
High-pitched crying (babies)	Bulging fontanelle (babies)
Drowsiness	Neck stiffness – Brudzinski's sign
Seizures	Kernig's sign
Fever	Photophobia (in older children)
Vomiting	Petechial rash (in meningococcal septicaemia)
Headaches	Papilloedema (rare)

A lumbar puncture is performed to examine the cerebrospinal fluid in order to identify the causative microorganism responsible. However, this should never be done if the patient shows signs of raised intracranial pressure, such as papilloedema.

In cases where the pathogen is not identified, a broad-spectrum antibiotic is used, such as cefotaxime. If *N. meningitides* is found, benzylpenicillin is the preferred antibiotic.

Deafness, cerebral palsy and subdural haemorrhages are possible serious complication of bacterial meningitis if appropriate treatment is delayed.

18. Causes of Learning Disabilities

Word List: cytomegalovirus; Down's syndrome; fetal alcohol syndrome; fragile X; galactosaemia; head injury; hypoxic ischaemic encephalopathy; hypoglycaemia; Klinefelter's syndrome; lead poisoning; meningitis; neurofibromatosis; phenylketonuria; Prader–Willi syndrome; Rett's syndrome; rubella.

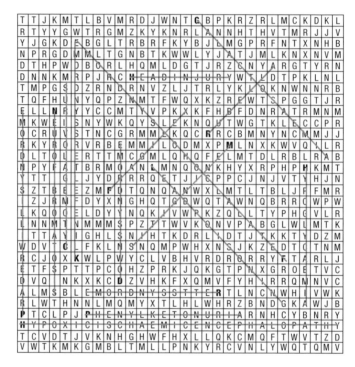

Classification	Disorders
Prenatal	Genetic – Down's syndrome; fragile X syndrome; Klinefelter's syndrome; Prader–Willi syndrome; Rett's syndrome; neurofibromatosis Metabolic – phenylketonuria; hypoglycaemia; galactosaemia Infection – cytomegalovirus; rubella Drugs – fetal alcohol syndrome
Perinatal	Head injury; hypoxic ischaemic encephalopathy; meningitis
Postnatal	Lead poisoning

An IQ of 50–70 indicates mild learning disability, whereas severe learning disability refers to an IQ of <50. Very severe learning difficulties are usually related to global developmental delay (see Puzzle 64).

19. Causes of Cerebral Palsy

Word List: birth asphyxia; birth injury; cerebral dysgenesis; cytomegalovirus; encephalitis; head injury; hydrocephalus; hyperbilirubinaemia; hypoglycaemia; hypoxic ischaemic encephalopathy; intraventricular haemorrhage; meningitis; non-accidental injury; rubella; toxoplasmosis.

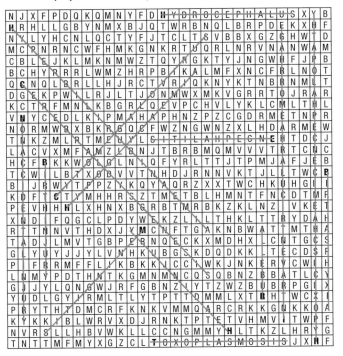

The most common causes of cerebral palsy are during the prenatal period, as opposed to the perinatal period, where birth injury and asphyxia are relatively uncommon aetiological factors.

Classification	Causes
Prenatal	Cerebral dysgenesis; cytomegalovirus; rubella; toxoplasmosis
Perinatal	Birth asphyxia; birth injury
Postnatal	Hyperbilirubinaemia; encephalitis; meningitis; head injury; non-accidental injury; hydrocephalus; hypoglycaemia; hypoxic ischaemic encephalopathy; intraventricular haemorrhage

20. Epilepsy in Childhood

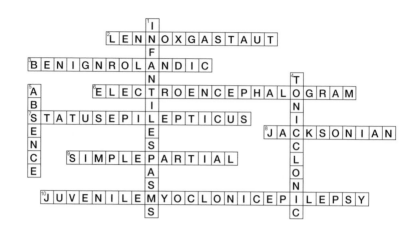

Epilepsy is the recurrence of convulsive attacks due to an electrical discharge from the brain. Diagnosis is mainly deduced from a thorough clinical history, from the child as well as an eyewitness of the seizure, which can then be confirmed by an electroencephalogram (EEG). Status epilepticus is prolonged or multiple convulsions without recovery of consciousness, lasting for more than 30 minutes.

Seizure	Comments
Tonic–clonic	Tonic phase (muscle rigidity), clonic phase (violent contractions) and unconsciousness
Absence	Loss of consciousness for usually <10 seconds
Simple partial	Consciousness and memory intact, affecting localized area of brain, e.g. frontal lobe (Jacksonian)
Complex partial	Consciousness and memory impaired
Lennox–Gastaud syndrome	In males 3–5 years old; myoclonic, absence and atonic seizures; associated with developmental delay
West's syndrome	In 4–6-month-olds; 20–30 infantile ('salaam') spasms
Juvenile myoclonic epilepsy	In puberty; mainly myoclonic, absence and tonic–clonic seizures
Benign Rolandic epilepsy	Onset 3–12 years old, lasting till 14–18 years old; tonic–clonic seizures; sometimes reading and learning difficulties

21. Antiepileptic Drugs

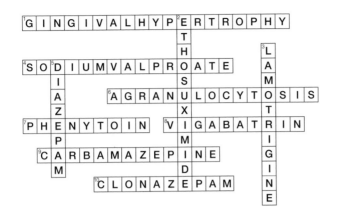

Drug	Comments
Sodium valproate	First-line treatment for generalized seizures; adverse effects include nausea, hair loss and liver failure
Carbamazepine	First-line treatment for partial seizures; adverse effects of drowsiness, diplopia, liver abnormalities and agranulocytosis (lethal and rare)
Ethosuximide	First-line treatment for absence seizures; adverse effects of abdominal discomfort and blood dyscrasia
Lamotrigine	Second-line treatment for general seizures; few adverse effects of rash, Stevens– Johnson syndrome
Vigabatrin	Treatment for infantile spasms; adverse effects of changes in behaviour, retinal damage
Phenytoin	Treatment for tonic–clonic seizures; adverse effects of chronic use include hirsuitism, gingival hypertrophy, ataxia, rashes and blood dyscrasia
Diazepam	Immediate intravenous treatment for status epilepticus; adverse effects of drowsiness
Clonazepam	Treatment of myoclonic seizures and alternative immediate intravenous treatment for status epilepticus; adverse effects of drowsiness

22. Causes of Cough

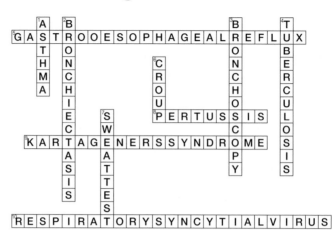

Disorder	Comments
Croup	Barking cough, stridor worse at night; can be life-threatening; mostly seen during winter
Pertussis	Bouts of loud inspiratory 'whoop' cough with apnoeic episodes followed by vomiting and epitaxis
Bronchiolitis	Infants 1–9 months old; caused by respiratory syncytial virus; peak incidence in winter; symptoms of wheezy cough, difficulty breathing and intercostal recession
Aspirated foreign body	Coughing or choking on foreign body (e.g. nuts) aspirated days or weeks earlier
Asthma	Cough with wheeze, worsens with exercise and at night
Tuberculosis	History of contact, weight loss and positive Mantoux test
Cystic fibrosis	Purulent cough, recurrent lung infections; diagnosed by the sweat test
Bronchiectasis	Profuse, foul-smelling green/yellow sputum
Gastro-oesophageal reflux	Cough-associated heartburn after eating
Kartagener's syndrome	Situs invertus (dextrocardia), chronic sinusitis and bronchiectasis (immotile cilia)

Bronchoscopy can be used to detect and remove an aspirated foreign body, such as a peanut.

23. Causes of Stridor and Wheeze

Word List: anaphylaxis; aortic aneurysm; asthma; bronchiolitis; croup; cystic fibrosis; epiglottitis; foreign body; gastro-oesophageal reflux; heart failure; laryngeal tumour; laryngospasm; maternal smoking; mediastinal tumour; pulmonary eosinophilia; rheumatoid arthritis; thyrotoxicosis; tracheal stenosis.

```
F X G B N Y J P R U O M U T L A E G N Y R A L
U U R L R T M L Y B R T G T V M N W B F K Z G
L L W H T R T S A T R B N F N H G M C W X J N
M F D E N A F G Y R X O N T W W K M M V J T
C E R A T C P C D R L N T J M H N T K N F K
N R U H H L L O K U N O C Z R B X L X F X O
A L O T Y E R B B Z M E G L H Q K R G G M P M
F A M F R A D M N L H G N O R K R P F B R S
Y E U A O L M M G T T M T A S B O C M N R T L
E G T S G F V K Q M N C R Y L L L P D A
C A L L O T X C E X M Y Y K M L A L U R D N
S H A U X E H P R R C C J T H N T S O T K R R
I P N R N X M O Q V Y D G A Q M X M X L E
N O E C O M N F D X C Y P N W C T O K N S T
C S T W O S T G T H P Y Z J N Q W B A T Q A
F E S P S V X T K D Y K L Y T D N R K K C M
H O A Z S E P I G L O T T I T I S V W A K J
I O J S Y M Y N Q H L V K G P C K M K Y D
L R D N J K N Y T Y T H H K G Y H H B X R N
I T E N Q M F K V X Q R X T M H L H D C N
A S M J L T S R R Z H K N T T G S M K R F W D
V A S H T H R H T R A D I O T A M U E H R J D
T G X J G C T M F C Y S T I C F I B R O S I S
```

Stridor can be defined as the sound heard on auscultation during inspiration indicating obstruction in the upper airways, mainly the larynx.

On auscultation, a wheeze is most markedly heard in expiration in the presence of an obstruction in the lower part of the airways, such as the bronchioles.

Causes of stridor	Causes of wheeze
Foreign body	Asthma
Croup	Foreign body
Epiglottitis	Cystic fibrosis
Laryngospasm	Gastro-oesophageal reflux
Tracheal stenosis	Bronchiolitis
Anaphylaxis	Heart failure
Laryngeal tumour	Pulmonary eosinophilia
Aortic aneurysm	Maternal smoking
Mediastinal tumour	
Rheumatoid arthritis	
Thyrotoxicosis	

24. Upper Respiratory Tract Infections

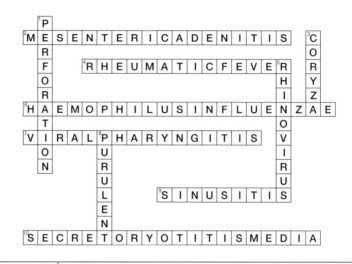

Disorder	Comments
Coryza	'Common cold'; commonest pathogens are rhinoviruses; symptoms include running nose, sneezing and nasal blockage
Viral pharyngitis	Features consist of sore throat, fever, inflamed erythematous pharynx and soft palate, and cervical lymphadenopathy
Tonsillitis	Bacterial cause in children over 5 years old; main pathogen is group A β-haemolytic streptococcus; clinical features of sore throat, dysphagia, fever, inflamed and enlarged tonsils, purulent exudate, cervical lymphadenopathy, sometimes abdominal pain (mesenteric adenitis); complications of post-streptococcal glomerulitis, rheumatic fever;
Secretory otitis media	Pathogens include *Streptococcus pneumoniae*, *Haemophilus influenzae*, or poor Eustachian tube ventilation; clinical features of ear pain, fever, hearing loss, inflamed tympanic membrane, which may perforate
Acute epiglottitis	Main pathogen is *H. influenzae* type b; features of sudden-onset stridor, fever, toxic appearance, dysphonia, dysphagia, dyspnoea, drooling
Sinusitis	Features include pain and tenderness in maxillary sinus with nasal discharge when infected
Obstructive sleep apnoea	Main cause is adenotonsillar hypertrophy; clinical features of snoring, apnoea, sometimes failure to thrive, poor academic performance, enuresis.

25. Lower Respiratory Tract Infections

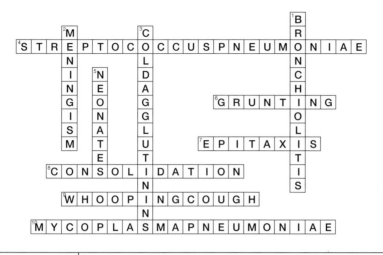

Disorder	Comments
Pneumonia	Pathogens – group B β-haemolytic streptococcus is the main cause in the neonate; *Steptococcus pneumoniae* is the commonest cause of lobar pneumonia; *Mycoplasma pneumoniae* affects schoolchildren Symptoms of initial fever, shortness of breath, cough leading to tachypnoea, grunting (suggests respiratory distress) on expiration, pleuritic chest pain and sometimes meningism and abdominal pain Signs of consolidation – dullness on percussion, reduced breath sounds, bronchial breathing Investigations include a chest x-ray, blood cultures, nasopharyngeal aspirate; cold agglutinins confirms *M. pneumoniae*
Bronchiolitis	Mainly in babies 1–9 months old; caused by RSV. Symptoms of coryza progresses to cough, dyspnoea, shortness of breath, feeding difficulties Signs of tachypnoea, cyanosis, subcostal and intercostal recession, chesty hyperinflation, diffuse fine crepitations, wheeze
Whooping cough	Caused by *Bordetella pertussis* Symptoms consist of 2 days of coryza, leading to spasmodic bouts of coughing with inspiratory 'whoop' – child goes blue, and severe episodes lead to epitaxis and subconjunctival haemorrhage; cough worse at night.

26. Asthma

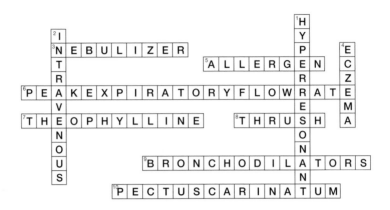

Asthma is a chronic reversible obstructive airway disease brought on by a specific allergen, infection, exercise and emotion.

Symptoms consist of episodes of shortness of breath, cough and wheezing. It may be accompanied by other atopic illnesses, such as eczema. On inspection of the chest, the patient may have a chest deformity known as pectus carinatum, which is suggestive of chronic airway obstruction. During acute asthmatic attacks, the chest will appear hyperresonant along with diffuse expiratory rhonchi heard on auscultation.

Peak flow expiratory rate can be used to confirm the diagnosis in children over 5 years old. However, in an acute attack, a chest x-ray is useful to reveal hyperinflation of the chest.

Type	Drugs
Relievers	Bronchodilators, e.g. salbutamol Ipratropium bromide
Preventers	Oral prednisolone (side effect – thrush) Theophylline Sodium cromoglycate

Intravenous hydrocortisone and intravenous aminophylline are administered in status asthmaticus if the child does not respond to bronchodilators delivered through nebulizers (in vaporized form) with oxygen.

27. Cystic Fibrosis

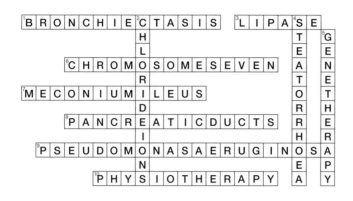

Cystic fibrosis is an autosomal recessive condition caused by a mutant gene on chromosome 7. The gene is responsible for coding the cystic fibrosis transmembrane regulator (CFTR) which transports chloride ions in the epithelial cells.

System	Clinical features
Respiratory	Recurrent infections present with purulent cough and wheeze; can lead to bronchiectasis Meconium ileus – intestinal obstruction with symptoms of vomiting, abdominal distension and delayed passage of meconium in first 2 days after birth
Gastro-intestinal	Obstructed pancreatic ducts leads to insufficient pancreatic enzymes, e.g. lipase and amylase, presenting with steatorrhoea and malabsorption Finger clubbing
Other	Cirrhosis Diabetes mellitus Infertility

Cystic fibrosis is managed by a combination of physiotherapy to break-up the viscous sputum in the chest and nutritional supplements to introduce pancreatic enzymes into the body. Antibiotics are required when respiratory infections emerge, such as *Staphylococcus aureus*, *Haemophilus influenzae* and *Pseudomonas aeruginosa*. Research is currently being undertaken into the possibility of gene therapy.

28. Murmurs

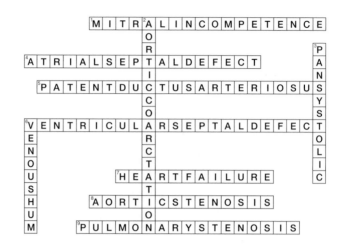

Murmur	Comments
Ventricular septal defect	Most common congenital heart disease; pansystolic murmur at lower left sternal edge, can radiate to the back
Atrial septal defect	Ejection systolic murmur heard at 3rd intercostal space
Patent ductus arteriosus	Continuous machinery murmur heard at left sternal edge
Aortic stenosis	Ejection systolic murmur at upper right sternal edge, radiates to neck and associated with ejection click
Aortic coarctation	Systolic murmur heard between shoulder blades, with weak/absent femoral pulse
Pulmonary stenosis	Systolic murmur at upper left sternal edge radiating to back, associated with ejection click
Mitral incompetence	Continuous murmur at apex, radiates to axilla and back

Pansystolic murmur occurs when the heart sound lasts throughout the entire systolic phase with equal intensity.

The presence of a third heart sound can indicate heart failure or can merely be a physiological occurrence.

A venous hum is an innocent murmur characterized by a low-pitched continuous sound heard below the clavicles. It can no longer be heard when the individual lies down.

29. Clinical Features of Infective Endocarditis

Word List: anaemia; anorexia; athralgia; cerebral abscess; clubbing; fever; headache; malaise; murmur; retinal infarcts; splenomegaly; splinter haemorrhages.

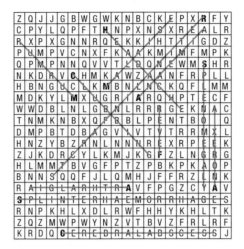

Infective endocarditis should be suspected in all children with a history of sustained fever and an audible heart murmur.

Symptoms	Signs
Anorexia	Retinal infarcts
Arthralgia	Anaemia (pale conjunctiva)
Fever	Clubbing
Headache	Murmur
Malaise	Splenomegaly
	Splinter haemorrhages
	Cerebral abscess

To prevent infective endocarditis, antibiotics need to be administered for any child with congenital heart disease before dental or surgical treatment.

30. Congenital Heart Disease

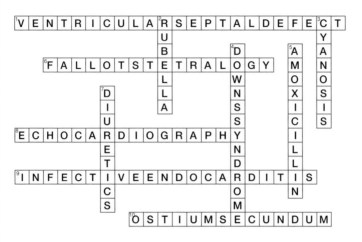

Disorders	Comments
Ventricular septal defect (VSD)	Most common congenital heart disease; symptoms depend on size of defect – can lead to heart failure in childhood
Atrial septal defect	Less common; two main types – ostium secundum defect (more common), and ostium primum; associated with Down's syndrome; complications of secundum consist of pulmonary hypertension, right-sided heart failure and stroke
Fallot's tetralogy	Combination of VSD, right ventricular hypertrophy, pulmonary stenosis and overriding aorta; main symptom is cyanosis from first year of life; during childhood, the child squats to overcome lack of oxygen

Infections (e.g. rubella), alcohol and medications (e.g. retinoic acid) are all aetiological factors in congenital heart disease.

An echocardiogram is performed to visualize and identify congenital heart anomalies. Other useful diagnostic investigations include a chest x-ray and ECG.

The management of heart failure includes diuretics, angiotensin-converting enzyme inhibitors and β-blockers.

In order to prevent children with congenital heart disease from acquiring infective endocarditis, amoxicillin is given prior to any surgical procedure.

31. Anaemia

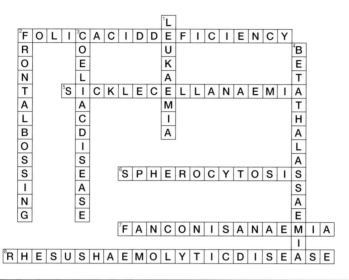

Disorder	Comments
β-thalassaemia	In those from the Mediterranean and Asia; features of severe anaemia, jaundice, short stature, hepatomegaly, face – frontal bossing and maxillary overgrowth
Sickle-cell anaemia	In those of African descent; features of anaemia, jaundice, vaso-occlusive crises (profound pain in long bones, back and chest, dactylitis) swollen hands and feet, and splenic infarction, which increases risk of serious infections
Spherocytosis	Mis-shaped erythrocytes; features of mild anaemia, jaundice, splenomegaly and increased risk of gallstones
Coeliac disease	Gluten-sensitive enteropathy; features of anaemia (iron-deficiency), fatigue, failure to thrive and steatorrhoea
Rhesus haemolytic disease	Rare; usually detected antenatally; features of mild anaemia, hepatosplenomegaly, respiratory distress in fetus, and can cause death; can be prevented by giving anti-D immunoglobulin to Rhesus –ve mother after birth of Rhesus +ve baby
Folic acid deficiency	More common in those with poor diet, alcoholics, and in pregnancy; features of fatigue, pallor and palpitations
Leukaemia	Features of pallor, purpura, hepatomegaly, lymphadenopathy and bone pain
Fanconi's anaemia	Pancytopenia with features of skin pigmentation, abnormal radius and increased likelihood of malignancy, in particular leukaemia

32. Bleeding Disorders

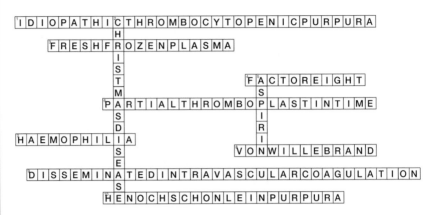

Disorder	Comments
Haemophilia	Haemophilia A due to deficiency of factor VIII; haemophilia B (Christmas disease) due to deficiency of factor IX; clinical features of prolonged bleeding after injury; in severe cases – haemoarthrosis in joints and muscles, can lead to arthritis in later life
von Willebrand's disease	Autosomal dominant; deficiency of von Willebrand factor; features of easy bruising, epitaxis, bleeding gums, heavy menorrhagia; in severe cases – bleeding into muscles and joints
Disseminated intravascular coagulation	Due to overactive clotting cascade; acute features of bleeding in various parts of body, e.g. venepuncture sites, soft palate and legs; chronic disease manifests as venous thromboembolism; treated with fresh frozen plasma (to replace clotting factors) and platelets
Henoch–Schönlein purpura	Symmetrical purpuric rash on buttocks and lower extremities, arthritis (knees, ankles), colicky abdominal pain and melaena; microscopic haematuria and proteinuria
Idiopathic thrombocytopenic purpura	Petechial rash, gingival bleeding, epitaxis, menorrhagia, intracranial haemorrhage (rare)

Partial thromboplastin time looks at the efficacy of the intrinsic and coagulation cascade. Aspirin and non-steroidal anti-inflammatory drugs should never be given to a patient with a bleeding or clotting disorder.

33. Malignancy I

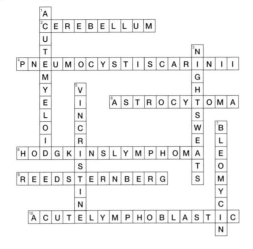

	Across the grid (filled letters)
1 (down)	AUTMYELOI... (AMYELOI)
2	CEREBELLUM
3	NGHSWEATS
4	PNEUMOCYSTISCARINII
5	VINCR...
6	ASTROCYTOMA
7	BLEOMYCIN
8	HODGKINSLYMPHOMA
9	REEDSTERNBERG
10	ACUTELYMPHOBLASTIC

Disorder	Comments
Acute lymphoid leukaemia (ALL)	Most common leukaemia in childhood; affects 3–6-year-olds; non-specific symptoms of malaise, fever, pallor, bruising, lymphadopathy and hepatomegaly; treated with chemotherapy and radiotherapy
Acute myeloid leukaemia (AML)	Associated with some genetic disorders, e.g. Down's syndome; symptoms of lethargy and lymphadenopathy; treated with more potent chemotherapy; prognosis not as good as ALL
Hodgkin's lymphoma	Affects young adults; symptoms of painless lymphadenopathy in neck; rarely 'B' symptoms of drenching night sweats, fever, weight loss and pruritis; diagnostic biopsy reveals Reed–Sternberg cells
Non-Hodgkin's lymphoma	Affects young children; often asymptomatic, depends on size of tumour – can present with lymphadenopathy
Brain tumour	Symptoms mostly due to raised intracranial pressure – vomiting, headaches and papilloedema; astrocytoma is the most common type, is likely to be found in the cerebellum and has a generally good prognosis

A common drug regimen to treat ALL is mechlorethamine, vincristine, procarbazine and prednisolone (MOPP). Bleomycin is another alkylating agent commonly given to patients with leukaemia; it has a serious side effect of nephrotoxicity. Immunosuppression is a consequence of chemotherapy, and specific infections, such as *Pneumocystis carinii*, should be treated with appropriate antibiotics.

34. Malignancy II

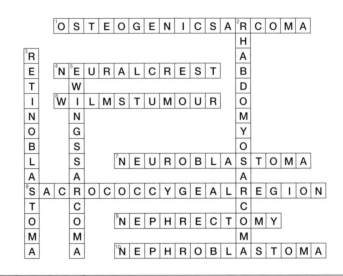

Disorder	Comments
Neuroblastoma	Tumour derived from neural crest cells, originating mainly from adrenal glands; affects mainly <5-year-olds; symptoms of large abdominal mass, weight loss and bleeding; increased levels of urinary catecholamines
Wilms' tumour	Also known as nephroblastoma; affects mainly 3-year-olds; typical presentation is large abdominal mass, but can also have abdominal pain, hypertension and microhaematuria; advanced metastatic cases can be treated with chemotherapy and nephrectomy
Retinoblastoma	Hereditary; absent red reflex, instead white pupils or squint; symptoms of severe visual impairment
Bone sarcoma	Osteogenic sarcoma is more common and affects younger children than Ewing's sarcoma; both present with long-bone pain precipitated by activity and localized swelling (in particular the humerus, femur and pelvis), or a fracture following a minor injury
Rhabdomyo-sarcoma	Tumour of the muscle or fibrous tissue; typical presentation is nasal and throat obstruction with blood-stained discharge or exophthalmus
Germ cell tumour	Originates from fetal yolk sac; most common site is sacrococcygeal region, followed by the ovary, testes and brain

35. Causes of Tall Stature

Word List: acromegaly; Beckwith–Wiedemann syndrome; congenital adrenal hyperplasia; Cushing's syndrome; gigantism; homocystinuria; hyperthyroidism; Kallmann's syndrome; Klinefelter's syndrome; Marfan's syndrome; maternal diabetes; obesity; precocious puberty and Soto's syndrome.

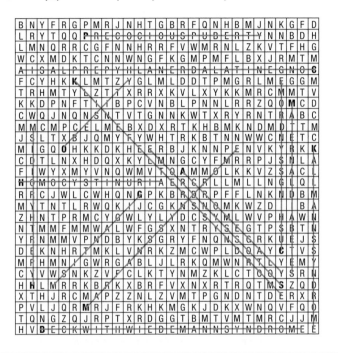

Cause	Disorders
Hormonal	Acromegaly; congenital adrenal hyperplasia; Cushing's syndrome; gigantism; hyperthyroidism
Genetic	Beckwith–Wiedemann syndrome; Kallmann's syndrome; Klinefelter's syndrome; Marfan's syndrome; Soto's syndrome
Other	Homocystinuria; maternal diabetes; obesity; precocious puberty

Note that the majority of children whose height is above the 97th centile are normal and there is no pathological cause.

36. Diabetes Mellitus

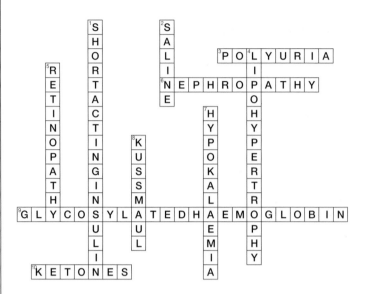

Timing of presentation	Clinical features
Initial presentation	Common – weight loss; polyuria; polydipsia; enuresis; recurrent infections Rare – ketoacidosis: vomiting, dehydration, Kussmaul breathing (deep laboured breathing)
Long-term Complications	Retinopathy; nephropathy (microalbuminaemia); neuropathy

The body reverts to the breakdown of fat to ketones when it is unable to metabolize glucose, which is due to the lack of insulin, and this results in diabetic ketoacidosis.

The diagnosis is primarily based on symptoms, the blood glucose levels being >11.1 mmol/L, glycosuria and ketonuria. Glycosylated haemoglobin levels are objective measures to confirm and also assess control over diabetes mellitus.

Drug management usually consists of a regime of short- and medium-acting insulin injected subcutaneously twice a day. Injection sites need to be rotated to avoid lipohypertrophy. The child and family need to be educated to administer the insulin, understand the dietary requirements and manage hypoglycaemic attacks. The main aims of treating the medical emergency, ketoacidosis, are rehydration (using normal saline), blood glucose control and electrolyte balance, in particular potassium levels (treating hypokalaemia – T-wave changes).

37. Causes of Hypoglycaemia

Word List: Addison's disease; adrenal cancer; alcoholism; breast cancer; congenital adrenal hyperplasia; diabetes mellitus; galactosaemia; glycogen storage disease; growth hormone deficiency; hyperinsulinoma; hypopituitarism; insulin; liver disease; Reye's syndrome; sulphonylurea.

Cause	Disorders
Metabolic	Glycogen storage disease; diabetes mellitus; liver disease
Hormonal	Addison's disease; adrenal cancer; growth hormone deficiency; hyperinsulinoma; hypopituitarism; congenital adrenal hyperplasia; galactosaemia; breast cancer
Drug-induced	Insulin; sulphonylureas; Reye's syndrome (aspirin); alcoholism

Hypoglycaemia is frequently defined as the plasma glucose levels being <2.6 mmol/L. It can be assessed firstly by using glucose-sensitive strips at the bedside, and then blood and urine samples need to be sent to the laboratory for accurate measurements.

38. Endocrine and Metabolic Disorders

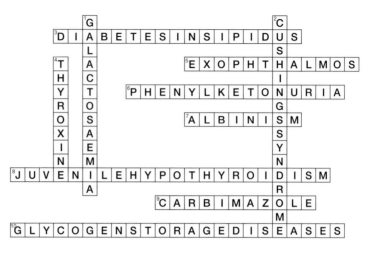

Disorder	Comments
Hyperthyroidism	Symptoms of restlessness, weight loss, diarrhoea and learning difficulties, ocular features are rare e.g. exophthalmos; treated with carbimazole, and β-blockers for symptomatic relief
Hypothyroidism	Congenital or acquired; juvenile hypothyroidism is an autoimmune disorder – more common in children with diabetes and Down's syndrome; if congenital hypothyroidism is left untreated, it can cause neurological complications; treatment includes thyroxine
Cushing's syndrome	Excess glucocorticoid, can be from chronic corticosteroid use; typical features of moon-shaped face, buffalo hump and raised blood pressure
Diabetes insipidus	Inability to produce ADH (cranial) or respond to ADH (nephrogenic); symptoms of polyuria and polydipsia
Phenylketonuria	Detected by the Guthrie test during neonatal period; if left untreated, results in global developmental delay and hypopigmentation (fair skin and hair)
Galactosaemia	Unable to metabolize galactose in milk products; neonatal jaundice can lead to chronic liver disease, coagulation defects and cataracts
Glycogen storage diseases	E.g. von Gierke's and Pompe's diseases; abnormal glycogen synthesis and metabolism; features of hepatomegaly, hypoglycaemia with further complications of cardiovascular disease and hepatic adenoma
Albinism	Abnormality in melanin synthesis; symptoms of depigmentation of skin and eyes and pendular nystagmus; increased risk of skin cancer

39. Causes of Neck Lumps

Word List: branchial cyst; cervical adenitis; cystic hygroma; dermoid cyst; infectious mononucleosis; leukaemia; thyroglossal cyst; lipoma; lymphoma; mastoiditis; mumps; sternomastoid tumour; thyroid carcinoma; thyroiditis; torticollis; tuberculosis; upper respiratory tract infection.

Cause	Disorders
Congenital	Branchial cyst; cystic hygroma; dermoid cyst; thyroglossal cyst; torticollis
Infection	Cervical adenitis; infectious mononucleosis; mastoiditis; mumps; tuberculosis; upper respiratory tract infection
Tumours	Leukaemia; lymphoma; sternomastoid tumour; thyroid carcinoma
Others	Lipoma; thyroiditis

The main cause of a swelling in the neck is an infection, in particular an acute upper respiratory tract infection that manifests as lymphadenopathy.

40. Leg Pain and Limp

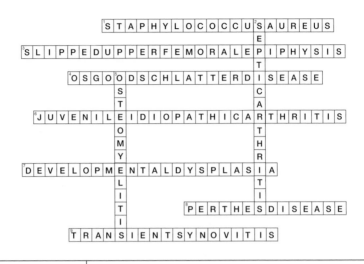

Disorder	Comments
Development dysplasia of hip	Dislocation of hip and acetabulum dysplasia; all neonates screened using Barlow's sign and Ortolani manoeuvre; if untreated, manifests as limp and waddling gait
Perthes disease	Mainly affects boys; intermittent leg or hip pain with a limp when walking; x-ray shows 'flattened' head in early stages, progressing to breakdown of bone
Slipped upper femoral epiphysis	Affects mainly obese 10–15-year-old boys; hip and knee pain for weeks/months with limp when walking, severe cases – cannot bear weight on affected limb; results in external rotation of leg when walking; x-ray shows displaced femoral head
Transient synovitis	Affects 3–10-year-olds; may be caused by viral infection, e.g. URTI; no systemic symptoms, only hip pain and limp
Osteomyelitis	Bone infection through recent trauma; commonest pathogen is *Staphylococcus aureus*; symptoms include pain and swelling of affected area and systemic features, e.g. fever and nausea
Septic arthritis	Serious infection of joints, can be caused by injury; symptoms of pain and warm swelling in joints and systemic features (fever, chills, nausea)
Juvenile idiopathic arthritis	Still's disease; presents with limp, flu-like symptoms and swelling of joints all over body, in particular knee, ankle and wrist; can progress to joint pain, stiffness and eventual joint damage
Osgood–Schlatter disease	Affects atheletic adolescent boys; symptom of pain below patella that worsens with exercise

41. Disorders of the Back

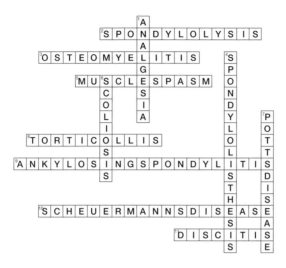

Disorder	Comments
Muscle spasms	Usually sports-related; caused by repetitive strain or trauma
Scheuermann's disease	Osteochondritis of the lower thoracic vertebrae in adolescents; clinical features of localized pain, tenderness and kyphosis
Spondylolysis	Stress fracture in pars interarticularis; usually affects adolescent atheletes; spondylolisthesis – vertebral bone weakens and shifts backwards, causing lower back pain and muscle spasms
Vertebral osteomyelitis	In a systemically ill child – insidious onset following septicaemic incident causing localized pain and tenderness, in particular when walking
Pott's disease	Complication of tuberculosis; back pain with fever, malaise and night sweats
Discitis	Infection of disc space; symptoms of severe back pain with insidious onset
Ankylosing spondylitis	Older adolescents affected; symptoms of back pain worse in morning, improve throughout day
Tumours	Benign and malignant
Systemic disease	Sickle-cell anaemia; renal abscess

Scoliosis is an abnormal lateral curvature of the spine. Its aetiology includes congenital, idiopathic and secondary causes, such as cerebral palsy. Torticollis, or a wry neck, is when a person's head is twisted and pulled to one-side.

The main treatment for back pain is analgesia, especially if it is muscular in origin.

42. Acute Rashes I

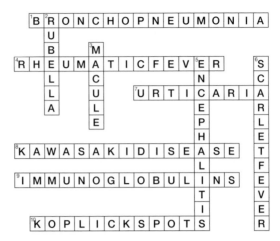

Rash	Comments
Rubella (German measles)	If acquired in pregnancy may cause fetal abnormalities; non-pruritic papular facial rash spreads diffusely, and lymphadenopathy
Measles	Prodromal phase of coryza, conjunctivitis, fever, cough and Koplick spots (white spots inside cheek); leads to diffuse maculopapular rash; complications of bronchopneumonia, otitis media and pneumonia; encephalitis (rare)
Scarlet fever	Coarse erythematous, maculopapular rash over head and neck and 'white strawberry' tongue; later face, hands and tongue desquamate; complications of rheumatic fever (rare in developed countries) and glomerulonephritis
Kawasaki disease	Mostly in Japanese children <4 years old; fever, rash, chapped lips and mouth, cervical lymphadenitis, erythematous hands and feet, which may peel; complication of coronary aneurysms, which can be prevented with administration of i.v. immunoglobulins
Urticaria	'Weal and flare' rash – transient itchy rash with raised papules surrounded by erythematous skin, usually due to allergic reaction, e.g. insect bite

A macule is a well circumscribed, flat (<10 mm diameter) lesion that blanches on pressure, e.g. found in measles and rubella.

43. Acute Rashes II

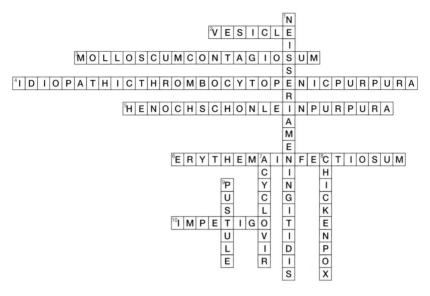

Rash	Comments
Erythema infectiosum (fifth disease)	Red facial rash ('slapped cheek' appearance) that progresses to maculopapular 'lace-like' reticular patterned rash on the trunk and proximal limbs with low-grade fever
Chickenpox	Pruritic rash of macules, papules, vesicles and crusting on trunk and face which spreads to scalp and limbs; complications of secondary infection of lesion and scarring, encephalitis, thrombocytopenia, pneumonia; immunocompromised treated with aciclovir
Meningococcaemia	Commonest cause is *Neisseria meningitidis*; initial symptoms of lethargy, headaches, vomiting, widespread purpuric rash within hours, +ve Brudzinski's and Kernig's signs; fulminant cases of high fever, chills, cyanosis and profound shock
Henoch–Schönlein purpura	Symmetrical purpuric rash on buttocks and legs; arthritis (knees, ankles), colicky abdominal pain; melaena; microscopic haematuria and proteinuria
Idiopathic thrombo-cytopenic purpura	Petechial rash, gingival bleeding, epitaxis, menorrhagia; complication of intracranial haemorrhage is rare
Molloscum contagiosum	Self-limiting; pearly white, wart-like lesions caused by a viral infection
Impetigo	Common bacterial skin infection on the face – vesicle with honey-coloured exudate causing crusting

A vesicle is a raised, serum-filled lesion (<5 mm diameter) seen in chickenpox.
A pustule is a raised lesion consisting of pus or clear fluid, e.g. in impetigo.

44. Causes of Purpuric Rashes

Word List: amyloid; aplastic anaemia; diphtheria; disseminated intravascular coagulation (DIC); Ehlers–Danlos syndrome; Henoch–Schönlein purpura; idiopathic; idiopathic thrombocytopenic purpura; leukaemia; Marfan's syndrome; meningococcal septicaemia; osteogenesis imperfecta; post-transfusion; psychogenic; quinine; steroids; rifampicin; systemic lupus erythematosus (SLE); varicella zoster.

Cause	Disorders
Low platelet count	Idiopathic thrombocytopenic purpura; leukaemia; DIC; aplastic anaemia; quinine; steroids; rifampicin; SLE
Normal platelet count	Henoch–Schönlein purpura; amyloid; Marfan's syndrome; Ehlers–Danlos syndrome; meningococcal septicaemia; osteogenesis imperfecta; diphtheria; varicella zoster; post-transfusion; psychogenic; idiopathic

Purpura is spontaneous bleeding into the skin. It is known as petichae when the extravasations are 1–5 mm in diameter and blanch on pressure. The appearance of deeper bleeding or bruising is referred to as ecchymoses, and is more commonly related to abnormal clotting or low platelet count (thrombocytopenia).

45. Management of Chronic Skin Disorders

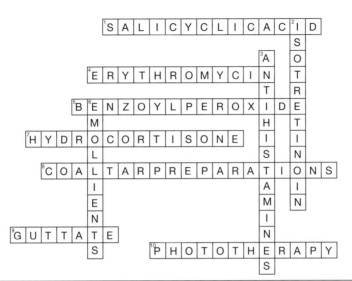

Disorder	Comments
Atopic	Emollients – used to hydrate and moisturize skin after bathing
Eczema	Topical mild steroids, e.g. hydrocortisone, for acute exacerbations – use sparingly Antihistamines – to relieve pruritis Topical antibiotics – if skin infected
Psoriasis	Coal tar preparations – for plaque psoriasis Salicyclic acid ointment – to remove plaques
Acne	Dithranol, corticosteroids, calcipotriol and retinoids are second-line treatments Benzoyl peroxide – topical keratolytic, bacteriocidal agent for mild cases Topical and oral antibiotics for moderate cases, e.g. erythromycin; tetracycline for moderate cases Oral vitamin A derivatives for severe cases, e.g. the retinoid isotretinoin – requires supervision from dermatologist

Guttate psorasis is the commonest type of psoriasis in children, with characteristic raindrop-shaped scaly patches on the trunk and upper limbs.

Phototherapy is an alternative to drug therapy for a range of chronic skin conditions, such as eczema, psoriasis and acne. Ultraviolet radiation is found to have therapeutic properties that suppress the immune system and decrease inflammation.

46. Causes of Acute Fever

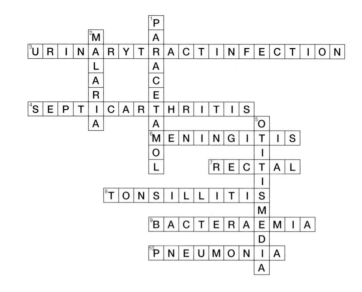

Disorder	Comments
Pneumonia	Viral – low-grade fever with dry cough and weakness Bacteria – high fever with rigors and productive cough
Tonsillitis	Fever with sore erythematous throat and white exudate on tonsils along with lymphadenopathy
Otitis media	Fever with ear pain, hearing loss and inflamed, erythematous tympanic membrane
Septic arthritis	Fever associated with a painful swollen joint
Urinary tract infection	Fever combined with frequency, enuresis and dysuria
Meningitis	Fever with vomiting, photophobia, headaches and neck stiffness
Malaria	Widespread in tropical and subtropical countries; fever, chills, nausea and symptoms of anaemia

A rectal thermometer reading provides a paediatrician with an accurate recording of the core body temperature.

Bacteraemia suggests bacteria present in the bloodstream and is often asymptomatic, unlike septicaemia, which does produce toxic symptoms.

A febrile child should be given antipyretics, such as paracetamol, to lower the body temperature.

47. Causes of Pyrexia of Unknown Origin

Word List: brucellosis; hepatitis; HIV; infective endocarditis; infectious mononucleosis; inflammatory bowel disease; leukaemia; lymphoma; malaria; Mediterranean fever; osteomyelitis; pneumonia; systemic lupus erythematosus; tuberculosis; urinary tract infection.

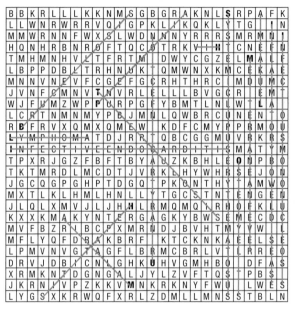

The aetiology of pyrexia of unknown origin is usually an infection, but occasionally it may be due to other causes, such as malignancy.

Cause	Disorder
Infective	Urinary tract infection; pneumonia; osteomyelitis; infectious mononucleosis; tuberculosis; malaria; brucellosis; hepatitis; HIV; infective endocarditis
Non-infective	Inflammatory bowel disease; leukaemia; lymphoma; systemic lupus erythematosus; Mediterranean fever

48. Shock

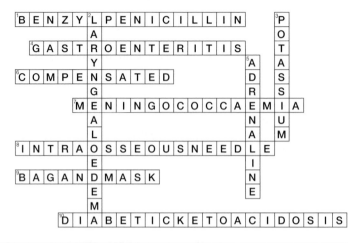

Type	Comments
Hypovolaemic	Causes include fluid loss, e.g. haemorrhaging, gastroenteritis and trauma
Anaphylactic	Symptoms include bronchospasm, laryngeal oedema causing hoarseness and features of shock; immediate treatment with i.m. adrenaline and i.v. hydrocortisone
Septic	Main pathogens are group B β-haemolytic streptococcus and *Neisseria meningitidis* (purpuric rash and neck stiffness – meningococcaemia), the latter of which is treated with benzylpenicillin if suspected
Diabetic ketoacidosis	In diabetes mellitus; treatment involves fluids for rehydration (i.v. saline); restoring and monitoring electrolyte balance (in particular, potassium), and i.v. insulin

In the first phase of shock, when it is considered to be compensated, the vital organs are still perfused; however, this can lead to decompensated shock, which can then progress to multiorgan failure.

The technique of the bag and mask is an effective way to deliver oxygen to children.

If there is difficulty finding intravenous access, an intraosseous needle can be inserted into the bone marrow cavity to reach the circulatory system.

49. Causes of a Coma

Word List: birth asphyxia; cardiac arrest; diabetic ketoacidosis; encephalitis; head injury; hydrocephalus; hypoglycaemia; hyponatraemia; intracranial tumour; lead poisoning; meningitis; Reye's syndrome; status epilepticus; stroke; uraemia.

G	D	C	S	U	G	I	T	P	E	L	I	P	E	S	U	T	A	T	S
X	G	L	N	M	Q	W	N	T	T	K	N	B	L	L	Y	M	K	T	M
S	I	S	O	D	I	C	A	O	T	E	K	C	I	T	E	D	A	I	D
C	L	H	T	B	L	Y	Q	M	B	M	S	M	Y	Q	E	B	D	K	M
A	J	F	H	G	F	P	S	Y	M	H	H	R	G	M	I	C	R	P
R	R	K	W	H	W	Z	T	T	K	V	N	M	O	R	F	Y	L
D	N	L	J	H	R	K	V	R	T	C	L	R	W	R	C
I	K	K	Z	T	T	Q	G	L	O	Q	N	W	B	V	D	H	T	U	T
A	F	T	R	D	T	N	N	G	R	O	K	J	X	F	N	A	K	J	Y
C	J	L	T	Y	R	L	A	S	H	L	E	L	T	Y	S	L	N	L
A	R	Z	L	N	N	Z	T	M	R	M	R	D	S	P	L	M
R	K	E	J	C	N	O	T	K	R	J	G	P	N	S	H	F	D	J
R	T	M	Z	A	N	O	T	D	G	V	A	W	W	L	E	Y	B	A	J
E	J	T	X	N	D	N	Q	C	L	G	K	E	R	L	Y	X	Z	E	Z
S	N	M	N	A	W	Y	L	X	Z	F	C	F	M	X	E	J	H	N
T	R	E	N	R	N	R	G	K	R	K	K	J	N	R	A	N	F	N
A	M	L	R	M	G	U	L	V	Z	T	K	N	X	R	A	L	F	H	V
M	M	K	W	N	G	L	K	E	N	C	E	P	H	A	L	I	T	I	S
T	R	U	O	M	U	T	L	A	I	N	A	R	C	A	R	T	N	I	N
N	G	B	K	H	Y	D	R	O	C	E	P	H	A	L	U	S	P	Q	W

Cause	Disorders
Infection	Meningitis; encephalitis
Metabolic	Hypoglycaemia; diabetic ketoacidosis; hyponatraemia
Drugs	Lead poisoning; Reye's syndrome
Trauma	Birth asphyxia; head injury
Others	Cardiac arrest; hydrocephalus; intracranial tumour; status epilepticus; stroke; uraemia

Metabolic disturbances are the main causes of a coma in children. As it is a medical emergency, the airway, breathing and circulation must be initially assessed followed by a neurological examination. This includes the Glasgow Coma Scale and the AVUP score, which assesses the level of consciousness of the child.

50. Poisoning

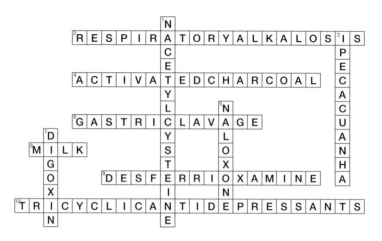

The crossword solution reads:

- ¹N
- ²RESPIRATORYALKALOSIS
- ⁴ACTIVATEDCHARCOAL
- ⁵N
- ⁶GASTRICLAVAGE
- ⁷D
- ⁸MILK
- ⁹DESFERRIOXAMINE
- ¹⁰TRICYCLICANTIDEPRESSANTS

Down words include: NACETYLCYSTEINE, IPECACUANHA, ACETYLSALICYLATE, NALOXONE, DIGOXIN, NALOXONE.

Management	Comments
Ipecacuanha	To induce vomiting in conscious patients
Gastric lavage	In cases of large quantities ingested or unconscious patients
Activated charcoal	Absorbant of chemicals, e.g. paracetamol; not effective in iron poisoning – use desferrioxamine for adsorption
Milk	Given in bleach poisoning
Antidote	Specific agents, e.g. naloxone for opiate poisoning and N-acetylcysteine in paracetamol poisoning

The symptoms of a patient with tricyclic antidepressant poisoning include arrhythmia, dilated pupils, dry mouth and drowsiness.

Common features of aspirin poisoning are vomiting, dehydration and hyperventilation which can consequently lead to respiratory alkalosis. This can develop into metabolic acidosis and eventually a comatosed state.

An individual who has taken an overdose of digoxin will present with cardiac arrhythmia and hyperkalaemia.

51. Non-Accidental Injury

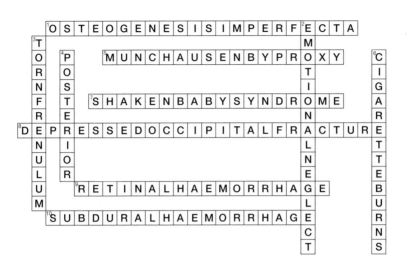

The crossword solution reads:

Across and down entries:
- OSTEOGENESISIMPERFECTA
- TORNFRENULUM
- POSTERIOR
- MUNCHAUSENBYPROXY
- EMOTIONALNEGLECT
- CIGARETTEBURNS
- SHAKENBABYSYNDROME
- DEPRESSEDOCCIPITALFRACTURE
- RETINALHAEMORRHAGE
- SUBDURALHAEMORRHAGE

Sign	Comments
Head injury	Subdural haemorrhage and retinal haemorrhage when the baby is shaken, e.g. shaken baby syndrome – with long-term neurological consequences
Fractures	Most commonly: posterior rib fracture from chest compression; depressed occipital or frontal bone fracture
Bruising	In particular trunk and face
Cigarette burns	Circular, clearly defined blisters with erythematous edges
Torn frenulum	As a result of blow to face

Munchausen by proxy is a fictitious disease, in which a carer – usually the mother – manipulates medical professionals into thinking that her child has an illness.

Emotional neglect can be defined as when parents do not show appropriate love or affection to their child. This can result in the child exhibiting signs of developmental delay and failure to thrive.

Osteogenesis imperfecta is an inherited disorder with clinical features of recurrent fractures, blue sclera and deafness. Repeated fractures have sometimes wrongly led doctors to mistake the disorder for child abuse.

52. Child Immunizations

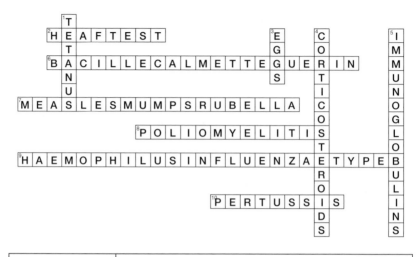

Immunization	Comments
Diphtheria, tetanus and pertussis	DTP triple vaccine – given at 2, 3 and 4 months of age; diphtheria booster given at 13–18 years old; tetanus booster at age 13–18 years or if child gets contaminated wound and was not vaccinated for 10 years
Haemophilus influenzae type b (Hib)	Given at 2, 3 and 4 months of age; to protect against *H. influenzae* meningitis and epiglottitis
Poliomyelitis	Live attenuated vaccine given in oral form; booster at 3–5 years old
Measles, mumps and rubella (MMR)	Given at 12–15 months of age; should be avoided if child known to have anaphylactic reaction to chicken eggs
Bacille Calmette–Guérin (BCG)	To prevent tuberculosis; given if tuberculin negative determined by the Heaf test; given at age 10–14 years

Taking corticosteroids is a contraindication to the administration of a live vaccine.

If a mother has chickenpox, the neonate is given intravenous immunoglobulins to prevent development of complications.

53. Maternal Infections and Drugs Affecting Fetal Development

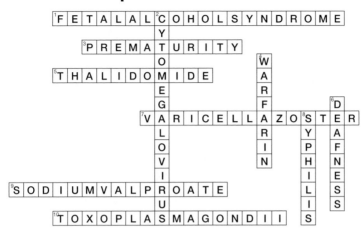

Infections / drug	Comments
Rubella	If acquired in first trimester can lead to deafness, cataracts and congenital heart disease in fetuses; preventable by MMR vaccine in childhood
Varicella zoster	Majority of mothers had chickenpox in past; can lead to cataracts, learning difficulties and skin scarring
Cytomegalovirus	No permanent damage in majority; fetus can develop deafness, microcephaly, cerebral palsy and learning difficulties
Toxoplasmosis	*Toxoplasma gondii* is spread through contact with cat faeces; majority of fetuses are unaffected; can cause retinopathy, hydrocephalus and learning difficulties in a few fetuses
Syphilis	Extremely rare; can cause ocular problems in babies; treated with parenteral penicillin
Thalidomide	Causes shortened limbs in fetuses; prescribed during the 1960s
Warfarin	Causes cerebral haemorrhaging in fetuses
Sodium valproate	Increased risk of fetal neural tube defects

Mothers who abuse drugs are more predisposed to delivering premature babies. Fetal alcohol syndrome can occur if the mother drinks alcohol excessively during pregnancy. A typical presentation includes microcephaly, learning difficulties, cardiac defects and dysmorphic facial features.

54. Birth Injuries and Asphyxia

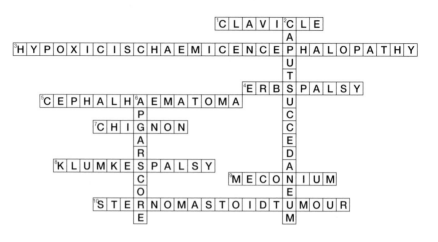

Birth injury	Comments
Fractured clavicle	Mainly from shoulder dystocia causing restriction of arm movement
Erb's palsy	Mainly from shoulder dystocia; affects upper brachial plexus; affected arm held in 'waiter's tip' position
Klumpke's palsy	Affects lower brachial plexus; claw hand and paralysis of intrinsic hand muscles
Caput succedaneum	Oedema crossing skull sutures of scalp, resolves in days
Cephalhaematoma	Subperiosteal bleeding within boundaries of skull sutures, resolves in weeks; occurs particularly following instrumental delivery or prolonged stage II of labour
Chignon	Temporary oedema of scalp post-ventose delivery
Sternomastoid tumour	Fibrous mass in sternomastoid muscle, following trauma, resolves in 6 months

Birth asphyxia means a lack of oxygen delivered to the baby's bodily tissues, including the brain, which can lead to the condition hypoxic–ischaemic–encephalopathy. Asphyxia leads to fetal distress, which is recognized by the combination of tachycardia or bradycardia, acidosis and the passage of meconium. The Apgar Score can be used to assess the general health of a baby 1 minute and 5 minutes post-delivery.

55. Complications of Preterm Babies

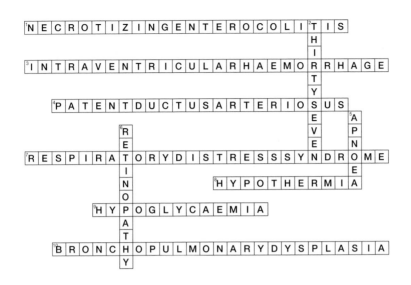

A baby delivered before 37 weeks of gestation is known as premature.

Complication	Comments
Respiratory distress syndrome (RDS)	Due to deficiency of pulmonary surfactant; signs of intercostal recession, tachypnoea, cyanosis and grunting; complication of pneumothorax, patent ductus arteriosus
Necrotizing enterocolitis	Gastrointestinal emergency; unknown cause; signs of bile-stained vomit, distended abdomen and bloody diarrhoea
Bronchopulmonary dysplasia	Chronic lung disease caused by high-pressure ventilation and high oxygen concentration; clinical signs of respiratory distress
Retinopathy	Due to high oxygen concentration; ischaemic retina leads to fibrosis, retinal detachment and possibly blindness
Intraventricular haemorrhage	Seen on cranial ultrasounds; can cause brain damage dependent on severity of haemorrhage
Hypothermia	Due to large surface area to body mass ratio and less body fat
Metabolic complications	Hypoglycaemia, hypocalcaemia

If the baby experiences episodes of apnoea, the aetiology needs to be investigated (see Puzzle 58).

56. Causes of Neonatal Jaundice

Word List: ABO incompatibility; birth trauma; biliary atresia; Crigler–Najjar syndrome; cystic fibrosis; cytomegalovirus; Dubin–Johnson syndrome; galactosaemia; Gilbert's syndrome; hepatitis B; meningitis; pneumonia; pyruvate kinase deficiency; rhesus disease; Rotor's syndrome; rubella; sickle-cell disease; spherocytosis; urinary tract infection.

Jaundice in neonates is a common medical compliant at birth; however, the majority of cases are benign and resolve within 1–2 weeks after delivery.

Type	Disorders
Unconjugated	ABO incompatibility; infections, e.g. urinary tract infection, pneumonia, meningitis; birth trauma; pyruvate kinase deficiency; rhesus disease; sickle-cell disease; spherocytosis; Crigler–Najjar syndrome; Gilbert's syndrome
Conjugated	Hepatitis B; congenital infection, e.g. rubella, cytomegalovirus; Dubin–Johnson syndrome; Rotor's syndrome; galactosaemia; cystic fibrosis; biliary atresia

57. Convulsions in Neonates

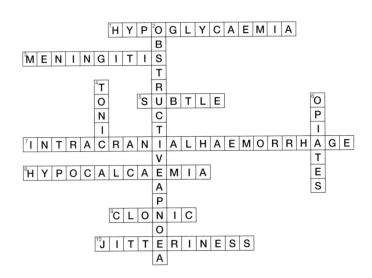

Cause	Disorder
Metabolic	Hypoglycaemia – can be prevented by feeding milk soon following birth
CNS	Hypocalcaemia – must always be considered Meningitis Intracranial haemorrhage – more common in preterm babies
Other	Opiate withdrawal Obstructive apnoea – blockage in airways Inborn errors of metabolism

'Jitteriness' is the term used for fine rhythmic movement precipitated by an external trigger, which ceases when the affected part of the body is held; there is no ocular involvement.

Prolonged normal activities, such as chewing, along with apnoea and eye deviation are known as subtle seizures.

A clonic seizure is slow rhythmic movements of an extremity or one side of the body, whereas a tonic seizure is defined as one extremity or one side of the body held in the extensor position, i.e. stiffening of the limbs or trunk.

58. Causes of Neonatal Apnoea

Word List: anaemia; asphyxia; beta-blockers; convulsions; gastro-oesophageal reflux; hypercalcaemia; hypoglycaemia; hypothermia; intracranial haemorrhage; kernicterus; macroglossia; meningitis; necrotizing enterocolitis; patent ductus arteriosus; pneumonia; sedatives; sepsis; tracheomalacia.

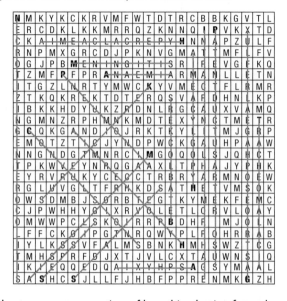

Apnoea is the temporary cessation of breathing lasting for at least 20 seconds.

Central apnoea occurs when there are no movements of breathing, and is due to neurological disturbances. However, in obstructive apnoea, the breathing movements are unaffected but the airflow is temporarily blocked.

Type	Causes
Central	CNS – asphyxia; convulsions; intracranial haemorrhage; kernicterus Infection – necrotizing enterocolitis; meningitis; sepsis; pneumonia Metabolic – hypothermia; hypoglycaemia; hypercalcaemia Haematological – anaemia Drugs – beta-blockers, sedatives
Obstructive	Gastro-oesophageal reflux Patent ductus arteriosus Tracheomalacia Macroglossia

59. Psychological Disorders in Adolescence

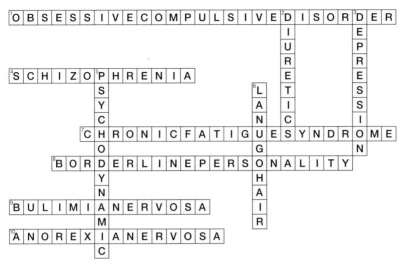

Disorder	Comments
Anorexia nervosa	Extreme restrictive eating to near-starvation; signs of severe weight loss, distorted self-image, emaciation, lanugo hair
Bulimia nervosa	Binge-eating and self-induced vomiting or ingestion of laxatives/diuretics; signs of oesophagitis, parotid swelling, dental erosion, fluctuating body weight, and metabolic imbalances, e.g. hypokalaemia, alkalosis
Depression	Signs of boredom, poor academic performance, social withdrawal, irritability, poor appetite, sleep disturbance, low mood and increased suicide risk
Borderline personality disorder	Tendency of individual to act impulsively, inducing maladaptive behaviour, e.g. acts of violence, suicidal threats and self-harm; difficulties controlling anger
Obsessive compulsive disorder	Features of recurrent, unwanted thoughts and repetitive, bizarre behaviour (e.g. hand-washing); comorbidity with other anxiety disorders, e.g. tics
Chronic fatigue syndrome	Post-viral infection, e.g. coxsackie B, signs of prolonged fatigue following exercise, myalgia, poor concentration and short-term memory
Schizophrenia	Onset in late adolescence; features include personality change, poor academic performance, social skills and psychotic symptoms, e.g. hallucinations

Psychodynamic therapy is a psychological technique unearthing deep-seated conflicts in order for the individual or family to deal with them more constructively in the future.

60. Substance Misuse

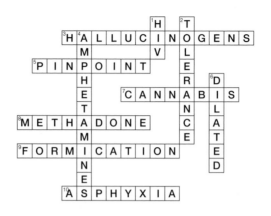

Drug	Comments
Solvent	Mainly adolescent boys and younger; sniffed from aerosols, glues; immediate effects of euphoria, excitement followed by drowsiness; adverse effects of asphyxia (from plastic bag), blurred vision, vomiting and facial rash; associated with high mortality rate
Cocaine	Snorted mainly; immediate effects of euphoria, increased concentration, dilated pupils; adverse effects of hallucination of insects under skin (formication), later depression and fatigue
Amphetamine	Immediate effects of increased energy, dilated pupils; adverse effects follow, including depression, anxiety and schizophreniform psychosis
Hallucinogen	For example LSD, angel dust, magic mushrooms; immediate effects of exaggerated perceptions, dilated pupils, hyperthermia; adverse effects include flashbacks, hallucinations and disorientation
Cannabis	Immediate effects of relaxation, enhanced mood; adverse effects of conjunctival irritation, psychoses
Heroine	Immediate effects of euphoria, pinpoint pupils; adverse effects of constipation, respiratory depression, drug dependence; withdrawal effects managed medically with methadone

Tolerance is the term used for the need to increase drug dose in order to achieve the same desired effect.

If there is any suspicion of the use of contaminated needles, the individual needs an HIV test.

61. Genetic Abnormalities I

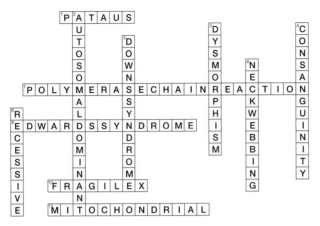

Type of genetic disorder	Examples
Chromosomal	Down's syndrome – trisomy 21 (see Puzzle 63) Turner's syndrome – absence of 1 X chromosome; features of neck webbing, widely spaced nipples, lymphoedema of hands and feet, coarctation of aorta Edward's syndrome – trisomy 18; features of low birth weight, learning difficulties, cardiac and renal defects, small jaw, overlapping fingers Patau's syndrome – trisomy 13; risk increases with maternal age; features of low birth weight, learning difficulties, cardiac and renal defects, small eyes, polydactyly
Autosomal dominant	Marfan's syndrome; Huntington's disease; achondroplasia; neurofibromatosis
Autosomal recessive	Cystic fibrosis (see Puzzle 27) Tay–Sachs disease
X-linked	Fragile X syndrome – mutation on long arm of X chromosome; features of learning difficulties, delayed speech and language, long face, protruding ears, prominent forehead
Mitochondrial	Leber hereditary optic neuropathy (maternal inheritance)

'Dysmorphism' is the term for abnormal anatomical developments, e.g. moon-shaped face, suggestive of a congenital disorder. The polymerase chain reaction is a technique used to amplify DNA samples to detect genetic disorders and identify viruses. The term 'consanguinity' can be defined as a person who marries an individual who has descended from the same blood ancestors; increases the risk of the offspring inheriting two autosomal recessive genes, which can result in an autosomal recessive disorder. A recessive gene is not expressed in a heterozygote.

62. Genetic Abnormalities II

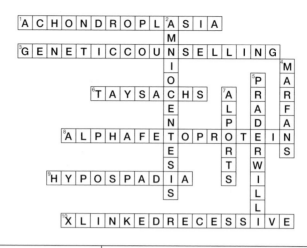

Disorder	Comments
Achondroplasia	Autosomal dominant genetic disorder; type of dwarfism – large skull, prominent frontal bone, short limbs, hydrocephalus and normal intelligence
Prader–Willi syndrome	Unexpressed or absent chromosome; features of obesity, short stature, developmental delay and hypogonadism
Marfan's syndrome	Elongated limbs, arachnodactyly, long face, cardiac defects, aneurysms
Tay–Sachs disease	Prevalent in Eastern European Jews; 'cherry red spot' at back of retina, hyperacusis
Alport's syndrome	Chronic renal failure, sensorimotor deafness, cataracts
Hypospadia	Urethral defect; can be associated with undescended testes

The 'triple test' to screen for Down's syndrome measures the serum levels of alpha-fetoprotein, unconjugated oestriol and human chorionic gonadotropin. Amniocentesis is a diagnostic test involving the extraction of amniotic fluid under the guidance of an ultrasound; used for karyotyping the cells of the fetus.

Haemophilia A and B are examples of X-linked recessive disorders in which only males are affected.

Genetic counselling assists individuals and families with the diagnosis and treatment of genetic disorders, as well as assessing the likelihood of their offspring developing an inherited disorder.

63. Complications of Down's Syndrome

Word List: Alzheimer's disease; brushfield spots; cataracts; clinodactyly; deafness; duodenal atresia; epicanthic fold; flat occiput; hypothyroidism; hypotonia; learning difficulties; myopia; narrow palpebral fissure; protruding tongue; respiratory infections; shortness; single palmar crease; squint; ventricular septal defect.

A combination of the features below suggests the diagnosis of Down's syndrome.

Abnormality	Clinical features
Face	Eyes – epicanthic folds; narrow palpebral fissure; brushfield spots; cataracts; squint; myopia
	Ears – deafness
	Flat occiput
	Protruding tongue
Limbs	Clinodactyly
	Single palmar crease
	Hypotonia
	Shortness
Other abnormalities	Learning difficulties
	Ventricular septal defect
	Duodenal atresia
	Hyopthyroidism
Complications in later life	Respiratory infections
	Alzheimer's disease

64. Causes of Developmental Delay

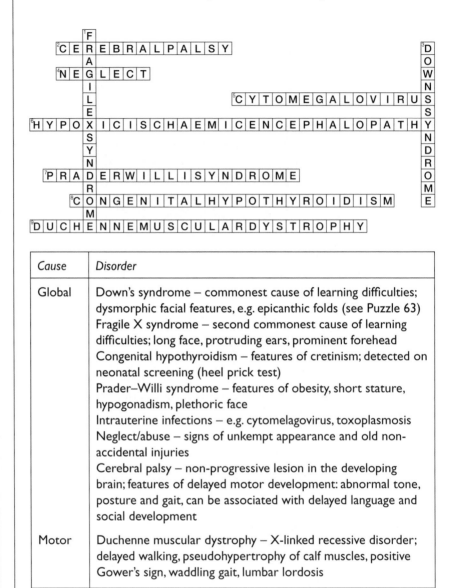

Cause	Disorder
Global	Down's syndrome – commonest cause of learning difficulties; dysmorphic facial features, e.g. epicanthic folds (see Puzzle 63) Fragile X syndrome – second commonest cause of learning difficulties; long face, protruding ears, prominent forehead Congenital hypothyroidism – features of cretinism; detected on neonatal screening (heel prick test) Prader–Willi syndrome – features of obesity, short stature, hypogonadism, plethoric face Intrauterine infections – e.g. cytomelagovirus, toxoplasmosis Neglect/abuse – signs of unkempt appearance and old non-accidental injuries Cerebral palsy – non-progressive lesion in the developing brain; features of delayed motor development: abnormal tone, posture and gait, can be associated with delayed language and social development
Motor	Duchenne muscular dystrophy – X-linked recessive disorder; delayed walking, pseudohypertrophy of calf muscles, positive Gower's sign, waddling gait, lumbar lordosis

Hypoxic ischaemic encephalopathy occurs as a result of birth asphyxia and can progress to cerebral palsy.

65. Emotional and Behavioural Problems

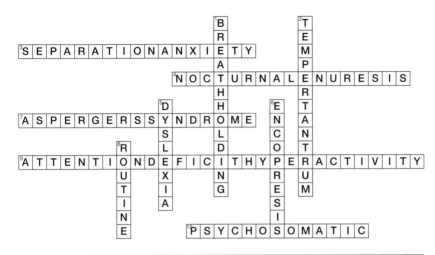

The crossword solution reads:

Across:
- SEPARATIONANXIETY
- NOCTURNALENURESIS
- ASPERGERSSYNDROME
- ATTENTIONDEFICITHYPERACTIVITY
- PSYCHOSOMATIC

Down:
- BREATHHOLDING
- TEMPRTANTRUM
- ENCOPRESIS
- DYSLEXIA
- ROUTINE
- ENURESIS

Disorder	Comments
Separation anxiety	Distress when infants (<6 months old) are not in the presence of an individual they are attached to
Attention deficit hyperactivity disorder	In preschool and early school; symptoms of poor concentration, poor attention, unable to sit still, restlessness and impulsive; can affect learning at school
Temper tantrums	Mainly preschoolers; angry episodes exhibiting aggressive and potentially destructive behaviour with lack of self-control
Breath-holding	In preschoolers; angry/upset child holds breath in expiration, leads to cyanosis progressing occasionally to temporary unconsciousness and convulsions
Nocturnal enuresis	Bedwetting; unlikely to have a psychological or pathological cause
Encopresis	Faecal soiling in >4-year-olds; caused by lack of toilet training, pathological constipation or psychological problems
Asperger's syndrome	Autism spectrum disorder; social impairment, repetitive stereotypical behaviour, normal language and cognitive development
Dyslexia	Difficulty in learning to read

A way to deal with the difficulty of sleeping in children is to introduce routine, i.e. making sure they go to bed at the same time every night. The term 'psychosomatic' suggests an underlying non-organic cause of a medical complaint.

66. Causes of Short Stature

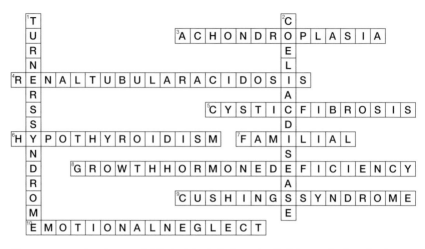

Short stature is when a child's height is below the 0.4th centile, but for it to be considered as pathological, the growth needs to be measured over 6–12 months and plotted on a growth velocity chart.

Cause	Comments
Familial	Look at family history – normal growth and within parental height range
Endocrine	Growth hormone deficiency – can be associated with lesions in pituitary gland; history of difficult birth and small genitalia Hypothyroidism – history of intolerance to cold, lethargy, pale yellow-tinged skin and constipation Cushing's syndrome – short stature with trunkal obesity and moon-shaped face
Chronic	Coeliac disease – associated diarrhoea and iron deficiency Cystic fibrosis – history of severe recurrent respiratory infections Chronic renal failure – e.g. renal tubular acidosis
Genetic	Turner's syndrome – features of webbing of neck, widely spaced nipples, lymphoedema of hands and feet Achondroplasia – disproportionately short limbs and large skull
Non-organic	Others – Down's syndrome, Noonan's syndrome Emotional neglect – look for signs of neglect, e.g. poor hygiene, and emotional abuse

67. Disorders of Sexual Development

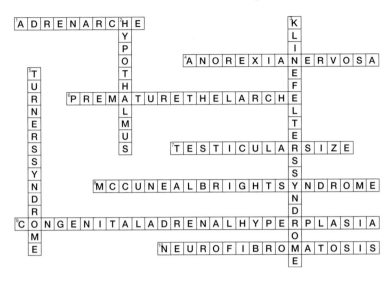

Disorder	Comments
Premature thelarche	Benign condition; early development of breasts (in females <2 years old)
Congenital adrenal hyperplasia	Autosomal recessive disorder; affecting males and females; female neonates have ambiguous genitalia, when older masculine features, e.g. facial hair, deep voice, no menarche; 2-year-old males may start puberty – enlargened penis, pubic hair; can be fatal if untreated
Klinefelter's syndrome	47XXY chromosomes; delayed or no puberty, features of long limbs, infertility, underdeveloped testicles and sometimes learning difficulties
Turner's syndrome	45XO chromosomes; features of neck webbing, widely spaced nipples, infertility, delayed sexual developments – small breasts, uterus and vagina, no menarche

Causes of precocious puberty include familial; premature thelarche; intracranial lesions, in particular within the hypothalamus; adrenal tumours; McCune–Albright syndrome; congenital adrenal hypoplasia; and neurofibromatosis. Typical features of neurofibromatosis include several benign growths beneath the skin along with early pubertal development.

Causes of delayed puberty include familial; pituitary disorders, e.g. tumour; chronic diseases, e.g. cystic fibrosis; Klinefelter's syndrome; Turner's syndrome; and anorexia nervosa.

The main distinguishing feature between true and pseudo-precocious puberty, e.g. congenital adrenal hyperplasia in males, is testicular size. In true precocious puberty, the testes are inappropriately large for their age.

The term 'adrenarche' is used to describe the early development of pubic hair.

68. Organic Causes of Failure to Thrive

Word List: cancer; cerebral palsy; cleft lip; coeliac disease; congenital adrenal hyperplasia; congenital heart disease; Crohn's disease; cystic fibrosis; diabetes mellitus; gastro-oesophageal reflux; heart failure; HIV; hypothyroidism; iron deficiency anaemia; lactose intolerance; renal failure; renal tubular acidosis; systemic lupus erythematosus; tuberculosis; Turner's syndrome; urinary tract infection.

Failure to thrive suggests poor physical growth and emotional development. It can be diagnosed by plotting the weight and height of the child on a growth chart on more than one occasion, and if either of these measurements falls below the second centile, it is indicative of growth failure.

System	Disorders
Respiratory	Cystic fibrosis; tuberculosis
Cardiology	Congenital heart disease; heart failure
Gastroenterology	Gastro-oesophageal reflux; coeliac disease; Crohn's disease; lactose intolerance
Neurology	Cerebral palsy
Renal/urology	Renal failure; renal tubular acidosis; urinary tract infection
Endocrinology	Hypothyroidism; congenital adrenal hyperplasia; diabetes mellitus
Others	Cleft lip; cancer; iron deficiency anaemia; Turner's syndrome; HIV; systemic lupus erythematosus

69. Neonatal Examination

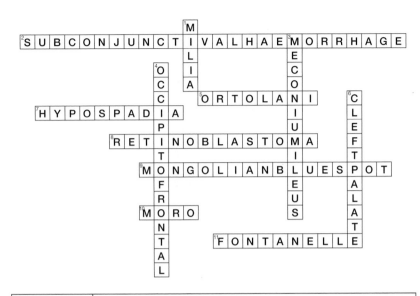

Examination	Comments
Head	Measure head size (occipitofrontal circumference) and palpate the fontanelle
Eyes	Check red reflex – negative in retinoblastoma; red patches can indicate subconjunctival haemorrhage
Mouth	Inspect roof of mouth (cleft lip)
Chest	Look for heart murmurs
Abdominal	Examine liver, spleen, kidneys
Genitalia	Look for clear definition of male/female Male – inspect testes and urethral meatus, for e.g. hypospadia
Hip	Otoloni manoeuvre to detect congenital dislocation
Nervous system	Check Moro reflex – tilt head back slightly, neonate extends arms, and then, brings them back towards the body
Skin	Mongolian blue spot – appears as bruising on lumbosacral area; more prevalent in Asian and African populations Milia – pearly white spots on nose and cheek

'Meconium ileus' refers to obstruction of the intestine and is a clinical manifestation of cystic fibrosis.

70. Developmental Examination

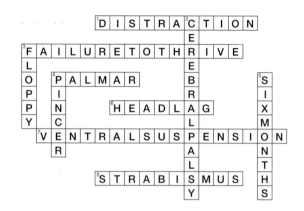

A developmental examination not only involves looking at an infant's gross
and fine motor skills, along with social and emotional development, but also
the child's speech, language, visual and hearing development. Key milestones
of development are assessed at different time intervals and compared
with the median age of skills achieved, in order to see whether the child is
developing at a normal, healthy rate.

Developmental examination	Comments (age)
Gross motor	Head control when pulled from sitting – poor control known as head lag (6 weeks) Sitting up without support (6 months) Ventral suspension – baby held in prone position shows head and limb tone, poor limb tone (floppy) Moro reflex – baby's head tilted backwards, arms extend, then brought back to body; asymmetrical response in cerebral palsy (birth to 4 months)
Fine motor	Palmar grasp – reaching for objects with whole hand (6 months) Pincer grasp – hold objects with 2nd finger and thumb (10 months)
Hearing	Distraction test – baby locates high and low frequencies without visual cues (6–9 months)
Vision	Cover test – testing for strabismus (squint)

'Failure to thrive' is the term used to show that a baby or child does not
meet the standards expected of growth.